A BAD REACTION

A MEMOIR

Sarah Bridges

Skyhorse Publishing

For my father, William Bridges, who guided me in writing and life.
And for Porter.

Skyhorse Publishing books may be purchased in bulk at special discounts for sales promotion, corporate gifts, fund-raising, or educational purposes. Special editions can also be created to specifications. For details, contact the Special Sales Department, Skyhorse Publishing, 307 West 36th Street, 11th Floor, New York, NY 10018 or info@skyhorsepublishing.com.

Visit our website at www.skyhorsepublishing.com.

10 9 8 7 6 5 4 3 2 1

Library of Congress Cataloging-in-Publication Data is available on file.

Cover design by Brian Peterson

ISBN: 9781634505376
Ebook ISBN: 9781510701472

Printed in the United States of America

NOTE FROM THE AUTHOR

Let me make something clear before you read this book: I believe in vaccines. My other children were inoculated and I received my own boosters before a trip to Africa. The discussion on vaccines has been twisted. We *can* be supportive of them *and* dedicated to improving their safety. These views don't imply an anti-immunization stance, in the same way that calling for safer airbags doesn't make us "anti-car." It is my belief that the suspicion of vaccines stems from the way in which the rare side effects have been handled.

1

4 MONTHS

Porter's high-pitched scream wakes us at midnight. I run to his room and pick him up. His sleeper is damp and his head flops to the side. His eyes are closed. I shout his name, but they stay closed. Brian grabs the phone and punches in the number for the hospital nurses' line.

"Hurry," I yell, even though he is dialing as fast as he can. He reaches for Porter, then hands me the phone, needing to hold the baby himself.

"Someone just answered," he says.

"What's the problem?" a voice on the other end asks calmly.

"Our baby has a fever and is listless. He was fine today," I say. "The doctor said he was perfectly healthy at his well-baby appointment this afternoon."

"Did he get his vaccines?" the nurse asks.

"Yes."

"It's probably the shots—fevers are typical after the DPT."

"But he isn't waking up."

The tone in her voice changes. "Get to the emergency room—I'll tell them you are on your way." I hear her, but I am frozen in place. This can't be happening.

I grab a blanket and press Porter to my shoulder, feeling his breath against me. *It's a good sign that he's breathing*, I tell myself. I hold him under my coat and run out to the garage. I am terrified. I've forgotten we also have a one-year-old daughter, Tyler.

Brian pulls her out of her bed and buckles her, still sleeping, into her car seat. He fumbles with the strap.

Go faster, I think.

He tightens the belt.

Go faster.

The freeway is empty as we barrel down it towards the hospital, the windows in the car cracked open for air. Porter lies on my lap with his eyes closed, and my legs feel hot under his body. We turn down Excelsior Boulevard, past the bar with the sign that reads THE BEST TIME OF YOUR LIFE.

A nurse meets us at the emergency room entrance in blue scrubs and tennis shoes. She has her arms stretched out to me so I hand her Porter and she carries him to an examining room. A man in the lobby sits hunched over and I wonder what is wrong with him. He hangs his head like he's lost someone, which maybe he did. I follow the nurse back to the examining room. She sets Porter on a bed and then she screams for help. I move forward.

"Not you," she says, and she pushes me back. "We need a doctor!" she yells and one runs in. I look past the two of them to Porter and see movement—I think he's waking up. But something is wrong.

His arms and legs thrash.

Shivers run through his body.

The doctor screams that he needs another doctor.

Porter begins a grand-mal seizure that lasts for ninety minutes. I am pressed against the wall, helplessly watching as a breathing tube is jammed down my son's throat. Porter lurches on the table while the nurse sticks a syringe of Valium into his arm.

After a minute the doctor turns to me and says, "Don't worry, we'll stop it. I'm sure about that. It's just that we may need to sedate him to the point that he'll quit breathing." In that instant, in that one sentence, everything I have taken for granted vanishes.

When the seizure stops, the testing starts—to discover whether an infection or virus caused Porter to become so sick. Tyler sleeps on two chairs pushed together in the corner. I've forgotten she is there. I should be worried about her too, but right now I can only think about Porter. Brian sits next to her, staring at Porter's motionless form. I stare too, but I can't sit still. I start to pace the floor. Every few minutes, Brian grabs my hand and tries to stop me but I just squeeze it, let go, and keep walking.

"He looks better," I tell Brian during one of my pit stops, trying to find something positive to say. I want to reassure him and have Porter back to normal again, go home, and start over. Brian pulls me towards him and I sit on his lap; he holds me there so I can't pace anymore. At 1:00 a.m. we are still sitting and staring; by 3:00 it is still the same but we both are frustrated because it feels better to be frustrated than scared out of our minds.

"How can it take ninety minutes to stop a seizure?" Brian asks too loudly and a nurse in the corner looks over at us.

"He's going to be okay," I whisper back. "Babies are tough. They always say that."

"They couldn't get the IV in—did you see all the pricks in his arms?" Brian says.

"At least they stopped the seizure."

"I don't want them stabbing him anymore with needles. I don't see how it helped anything."

"They said they need to do a blood test every few hours to check for infection."

"They also said they could stop the seizure and you saw what happened."

"At least he's okay now."

Porter takes a deep breath and moves his leg slightly. The nurse says he'll be asleep for hours—maybe even days, considering all of the drugs he received. I glance at the stack of magazines on the shelf next to me, wondering, *what am I supposed to do in the meantime—read* Glamour*?*

At 4:00 a.m., Porter's pediatrician, Dr. Amit, appears. She is hurrying into the examining room without taking notice of us. She wears sweatpants with winter boots, her hair pulled back in a rubber band. When she spots us she comes over and asks, "What happened?" She says it stridently, like we did something wrong. It makes me mad because I feel the same.

"I have no idea," I say, my voice sounding more defensive than I want it to. "You saw him this afternoon at his well-baby checkup—you said he was totally healthy."

"He was healthy," she says. "It's very strange."

She turns to the counter and opens a chart, then says, "The ER doctor called me and said Porter was extremely ill. I just don't understand how this happened so fast."

Brian and I walk over to Porter's bed. The nurse taking his pulse says under her breath, "You don't see that every day in the HMOs—a pediatrician coming from home in the middle of the night."

Our pediatrician goes down the hall to grill the other doctor about what exactly transpired. She doesn't understand what is wrong and demands to see Porter with her own eyes. Brian and I shift positions and stand next to the bed for an hour. Another hour passes after that. My legs are asleep, but I don't care.

"Do you want to lie down?" Brian asks.

"I can't. Why don't you try? The nurse said there's a couch around the corner."

"I can't do it either."

Instead, we stake our seats beside Porter, each of us touching an arm or a foot. Nurses come in and out. Doctors come in and out. Porter is motionless. *I don't know if I can stand this*, I think to myself.

They check monitors and medication levels. They stop to put a hand on Porter's forehead. I wish they wouldn't touch him, but I don't say anything. My hope creeps up with each passing hour without another seizure—just a little at first, then more. I find myself mulling about how this could have turned out. I start reframing my luck in terms of what didn't happen to my baby instead of what did. I hold Brian's hand—it feels warm and I think that everything is going to be all right as long as I hang on to it. Then everything is all right—by 9:00 a.m. all of Porter's tests are complete: no infection or virus.

After the tests, the doctors believe that Porter will be fine. He had a bad reaction, they say. He suffered a rare side effect to the Pertussis vaccine that causes seizures in some children and brain injury in a few others. But the brain damage is so rare they tell us not to think about it. I can't think of anything else.

Porter awakens in one piece and seems alert, but beyond that we are guessing.

The day after his seizure, he is still at the hospital for observation. The doctor asks, "Does he still do the same things he did before the reaction?" I stand there with my mouth a little open, speechless. I can't remember what a four-month-old does.

"Let's go home," Tyler says when she wakes up. She slept here too and looks tired. She puts on her coat and stands by the door.

"Porter has to stay here for a little while," I tell her, and she takes her coat back off. Brian and I huddle in the hall and decide to drive her to day care so that everything stays normal. Even though, right now, nothing is normal.

Brian and I sit in Porter's hospital room for three days straight. There is a rocking chair and a table with a Styrofoam pitcher. The crib has tall metal bars and looks like a jail cell. We trade off taking breaks. One afternoon I go down to the parents' lounge to flip through an issue of *Coastal Living*. I watch a father bend over a tiny refrigerator, trying to shove a take-out container between a dozen others. One falls out and noodles spill on the floor; he scoops them up and puts them back in the box. All the containers are indicators of the waiting time of parents before us.

My defenses are down. All of us parents are trapped in a no man's land.

A woman next to me appears to be glued to *Oprah* on the television suspended from the ceiling, but then I notice she's glued to the commercials too. As I turn the pages of my magazine she starts talking, "Why are you here?"

"My son had a seizure. What about you?"

"Our daughter was hit by a car. She's still unconscious, and her father won't see her." She takes a breath and speeds on, and she reminds me of Road Runner in that cartoon I watched as a kid. At any moment, I expect to hear a beep-beep. "He just can't bring himself to look at her that way. He thinks he's got to remember her exactly like she was—you know, the normal color before she was bruised. She'll wake up though. Another girl in St. Paul came out of her coma last year when they wheeled her outside and let her horse sniff her face. It could happen."

I nod my head in a way that might mean yes and might mean no but really means it's probably best if we just watch television.

"It could happen," she says again and I nod my head again.

I stare blankly at the pages in front of me, hoping she'll stop talking. I replay my conversation with the doctor after Porter's seizure ended. He told me that Porter might have epilepsy and said, "There's a guy in the NFL right now with seizures—he never misses a game." I know it was meant to cheer me up, but it made me feel worse. I picture Porter twitching on the table in the emergency room. I can't stop seeing it.

I go to Porter's room and he is asleep. Brian is back from retrieving Tyler at day care and I find her under Porter's crib playing with a plastic bedpan. Brian is bent next to the bed trying to coax her out with *Goodnight Moon*.

She shouldn't play with a bedpan, I think, but I don't say it because I can't remember why it matters. Tyler holds her arms out to me and I pick her up. She puts her head on my shoulder. She is soft and warm and I squeeze her hard until she pushes against me and says to put her down.

The nurse tells us to get dinner while we can, so I put Tyler on my hip and we walk down to the elevator at the end of the hall. A woman in a hairnet stands by the door pushing a cart with tiny vials of liquid. She is wearing purple gloves and waves at us with plastic fingers.

Tyler peers into a tube. "Why does she have all that blood?"

"She's doing tests, honey." It seems like the right answer, but my voice sounds strange.

"Mom—is Porter dead?"

I look at her to see if she is serious. I wish I could make her take it back. It strikes me that I am probably damaging Tyler through this whole experience. Maybe I'm exposing her to things she shouldn't see—like dragging a two-year-old to an R-rated movie.

"No, he's just sleeping," I finally answer.

Tyler smiles and says, "Okay," then jumps as the elevator goes down.

Someone said there is a McDonald's through the underground tunnel that links the children's hospital to the adult facility. We walk silently through the windowless corridor, past the signs for the asthma support group. One of them reads TROUBLE CATCHING YOUR BREATH?

The restaurant beckons ahead—a Ronald McDonald mannequin smiling with his hands on his hips. We line up behind a mother and her two boys. She digs in her purse and her kids hit each other; she says to stop it and they do. The boys then lie on the floor and she tells them to get up. She grabs their dinner and they follow her to a booth.

I scan the menu. "What do you want?" I ask Brian when it's our turn.

"I can't believe this happened," he says.

"He's going to be okay," I say quickly. "The doctor said it was a fluke."

"He said it's probably a fluke."

Tyler grabs a handful of straws and pushes them down her pants. "Look!" she says, as she points at them.

"Don't do that Tyler," I say. "What would you like to eat?"

"Chicken McNuggets," she responds, following the straws with a ketchup packet.

"I'll have that too, Brian. Porter will be okay. We just need to get him home." I say it with certainty because I'm sure it's good to be confident. *Porter's had a bad thing happen*, I think, *but we are already out of the woods*. I want to get back into our normal routine and I mentally roll through the days ahead. It is Sunday, and if Porter comes home the next day (which they say he will), Brian can go back to teaching and a week or so later I will resume classes and get going on my dissertation. Porter and Tyler will go back to their in-home day care, and we'll move past this in no time. We're practically home free.

Brian slides into the booth with us and hands me a tray of food. I look at his face and think to myself, *we dodged a bullet*. I can use what happened to Porter as a wake-up call. I watch Brian with his arm around Tyler and try to think of all the things that make me grateful. I look at Tyler, eating the chicken pieces one at a time. The straws she pulled out of her pants are on the table next to her in a pile. I try to freeze this moment by telling myself that I will stop packing our days so full that I don't have time to sit in the backyard and play with her. I have never even thought about the fact that I am lucky to have two healthy children. I look at Brian and Tyler and tell myself that I won't let it go back to being the same. I sit still for the first time in a long time and everything catches up with me; I feel like crying or laughing or maybe both. I slouch in the plastic booth, tapping my foot under the table, and watch my husband and daughter eat french fries.

As I stare at them I allow myself to drift away, remembering the trip we took to the Black Hills of South Dakota last summer. It was before we had Porter, before the seizure. It's hard to remember what that time must have felt like. Brian and I took the trip with the idea of buying a piece of property, lowering our expenses, raising vegetables, and slowing down. It would be a home we'd create over time. Brian knows how to build things—knows it in that intuitive, never-took-a-class way that allows him to wire outlets and install showers. We went west, chasing a dream that we could get something cheap with a few acres—something that needed work. We would get our hands dirty and turn it into a place we wanted.

This plan grew partly from our draw to rural spaces and partly from an idea that we could slow down and live more purposefully. One afternoon on the trip, we stopped at a tiny park at the base of a mountain and looked through a local real estate guide.

"It's amazing what you can get out here for $50,000," I said, pointing out a picture of a plot of five acres with a house and barn. There was a waist-high fence visible in the front. Brian and I were sitting on a wooden bench, old and full of splinters, a lone toddler swing beside us swaying in the breeze. There was no bright-colored plastic play equipment like in Minnesota; this park looked like it had been lifted straight out of my childhood. It was gritty and sturdy. It was dirty and charming and I loved everything about it. In the distance, the mountains were spotted with trees and shaded darkly. Even the field beside the park shimmered in the breeze. I kicked the sand under my feet and took a deep breath.

"We could even get a horse," I rattled on, thinking about my childhood in rural California and our obese quarter horse named Nipper. He lived in a pasture at the end of our driveway. All he did was eat and refuse to exercise.

"It's just the job thing we'd have to figure out," Brian said, sighing in the way he always did when we didn't have an answer to our problem. Brian was tired of teaching high school, sick of the treadmill of hourly classes, the endless papers to correct, the teenaged attitudes, the same problems year after year.

Brian and I had different childhood experiences, which gave us dissimilar outlooks on life. My life had been easy and happy: a childhood spent living in a California commune, picking apples and raising chickens, and family trips to Europe. Brian's life was less full of ease: He was a third-generation South Dakotan and an altar boy at the local Catholic church. He attended college and graduate school on a wrestling scholarship and spent weekends packed into the athletes' van driving from meets to seedy hotels. He starved himself on Thanksgiving to meet weight requirements.

His first year in college he got married, and then there were more wrestling meets and more bad motels, and raising two toddlers to top it off. He and his wife divorced after seven years, though they remained friends, and coparented their children in a way I admired. When he told me his story, I thought, *I can make up for the things you've missed out on. It is time that you have a slower pace. I can make you happy, just watch.*

We'd gotten very specific when we talked through our Black Hills plan. The conversation signaled a deeper need in Brian that I didn't recognize at the time. His reserves were low. He anticipated our future family with a yearning to shift the gears and go through parenting with more time and space this go round. He envisioned a peaceful pace instead of balancing the family time in the cracks and spaces left by unrelenting work. I liked the idea. I liked the conversation about how we would do it when we lived on that land.

"There've got to be jobs here. Maybe I can find a research role at the university," I said, even though I didn't want a research job; it was just the most obvious thing I could do with my graduate degree.

"Or maybe one of us could work and the other could stay at home," Brian replied. "I bet we could pull it off out here."

I nodded because I knew this sounded good to Brian, though not so much to me. Our second baby was due in two months and we already knew this one was a boy. I turned to the real estate booklet and scanned the photos on the back.

"Here's a four bedroom with a work shed." I held it up for him to see. "You could use that while you fixed up the house."

A group of kids rode past on banana seat bikes, three little girls pedaling slowly down the street. I thought about the pace here: the small towns and paint-chipped barns. I knew I was romanticizing the place, because it represented something more than the town to me.

I handed the brochure to Brian and lifted Tyler onto the swing. As I pushed it, her feet tapped my stomach and I pretended to be bounced backward.

"Baby jumped," she said, pointing to my belly.

"You made him jump high," I said.

"Tyler's sister," she added with a smile.

"Actually, he will be Tyler's little brother."

"No brothers!"

"We'll see," I said in a noncommittal way, knowing that I usually lost these debates and I'd better wait until I could prove it.

We stay in the McDonald's for an hour, eating ice cream sundaes after our chicken nuggets and watching Tyler touch the Ronald McDonald doll to see if he's real. When we finish, Brian prepares to take Tyler home since we don't have family in town and one of us has to get her to bed.

"Mommy *and* Daddy at home," she exclaims as we leave. "You said we'd always be together."

I do say this to her often and of course mean that our family will never split up. Tyler raised the question the week before when one of her friends at day care announced her parents were divorcing. I want to clarify but it seems inappropriate to raise the discussion that we aren't divorcing when she isn't asking. Besides, at three years old, she is the most literal person I know.

"We'll always be together," I say. "Just for tonight I'll be at the hospital. Besides that it will be always."

Both Brian and I want to stay, but we agree that I am the one most needed at the hospital in case Porter is able to breastfeed. We agree to this even though I know that Brian is thinking what I am thinking: that Porter probably won't wake up anyway. I return to his room and find him asleep. I climb into my cot, close my eyes, and wish I could sleep.

At 5:00 a.m., Porter is awake and smiling. He rolls over and bangs the bars of his crib, then settles down and goes back to sleep. I study him lying there on his stomach with his butt in the air, breathing lightly as a monitor next to him flashes his heart rate. Looking at him it feels like I am staring at a scene that could be a normal night at home, minus the machines and tubes. He looks peaceful and—above all else—normal.

I walk down the hall to the snack room. I am not hungry, but I'm dying to eat. Then I go back to Porter's room and lie next to him on my cot, drinking bad coffee and watching *The*

Today Show. I'm glued to Katie Couric. She is talking with a guest about the secret to a good soufflé and I focus on their dialogue like I am memorizing a language. *This is all I have to do*, I tell myself, *keep my mind on Katie and egg dishes and everything will be all right again.*

At 7:30 a.m., on our third day at the hospital, an intern comes in with a clipboard. Each morning we meet a new intern, and each time we run through events from the preceding two days. Was this his first seizure? Any history of epilepsy in the family? Allergy to drugs? Symptoms we'd noticed before he'd come to the hospital? I answer no to all of the questions, trying to smile, waiting to ask (as I have every doctor I've met so far) whether the seizure will cause permanent problems.

She glances down at her clipboard, "It can cause some losses—but it may not."

She's an intern. She doesn't really know the answer, I say to myself. Everything about the woman bugs me—her hair, her voice, her white clogs. I know I am being defensive, but I can't stop myself. I still hate her. As we finish talking, Brian and Tyler arrive and sit beside me as I balance Porter on my lap to feed him.

"He seems completely normal," I say, more to myself than anyone in particular.

"How did you sleep?" Brian asks, setting my change of clothes on the floor by the rocking chair.

"It was pretty quiet. How about you guys?"

"Tyler zonked out in the car before we left the parking lot," he says.

Porter finishes eating and I lift him up, breathe in the smell of his head. In the hours that follow, Tyler, Brian, and I play Chutes and Ladders, then I chase Tyler down the hall, and then we sit some more. Porter takes a long nap after lunch. His progress continues and by the end of the day he is allowed to go home.

In the discharge meeting the doctor says he believes that the seizure is a one-shot deal. "There's no reason to assume that he suffered any residual damage," he tells us, shifting from leg to leg. I wonder if he is nervous or if he just can't hold still. We sign the exit papers and we're free to go. We bundle Porter into a snowsuit and buckle his baby seat into the car. We drive away.

When we get home, I stand in the doorway to the kitchen and take in the scene. The garbage can stinks, and as I survey rotten fruit and dirty dishes I've never felt happier in my life. Brian puts Porter in our baby carrier as he picks up the living room, while Tyler helps me with the laundry.

I open the washer and she grabs my hand saying, "I do it." She smiles at me and I notice for the first time that she has on her Halloween tiara. We separate the lights and darks, sifting through the pile for any stray baby booties.

Brian sticks his head down the stairs into the basement and says, "Porter's sleeping in his car seat in the dining room. How about a pizza?"

"Just cheese," Tyler responds as she adjusts her tiara. "And crust."

"I already called—I'm going to go grab it." He gets ready to leave.

"I'll make some hot chocolate," I say, seeing the surprised look on Tyler's face. We never have hot chocolate and pizza. But tonight is special, more like a party. I pick Tyler up and carry her into the kitchen. I hear Brian's car back out of the driveway as we mix Hershey's syrup into the pan of milk. I look at Porter sleeping a few feet away and give Tyler an impromptu hug. Everything is going to be all right.

After we finish dinner and put the kids to bed, I take a long hot bath to try and relax. When my skin is too hot, I climb out of the water and run to my room, stopping outside the kids' room to listen for noises. It's quiet. I dart into bed and stretch my bare legs against the cool sheets, then rub against Brian's legs to feel their warmth.

I want to go back.

That is my first thought when I awaken at 5:00 a.m. I am wistful, thinking of the trip we took with my parents and sisters to Mexico a month before the hospital. We spent the days on the beach in front of the hotel, under thatched umbrellas.

I play out the scene in my mind. Tyler fills a pail and Brian sits with Porter on his lap. He is smiley and wiggly. My mother nicknamed him "Chuckles" because he grins at everything he sees.

"He's so easy," my mother says about Porter, who's looking at me. "He's obviously very secure in his attachment." My mother can't help these comments she makes. She is a psychotherapist and sees human behavior in 3-D. I expect the observations, but Brian looks puzzled. I still need to translate for him. I mouth the word "later," and he smiles like he gets it and my mother smiles back, sure that he does.

"They don't mean to eat people," I hear her say a minute later, engrossed in a deep conversation with Tyler—something about sharks. Tyler's eyes are big and I wonder what else my mother said because it could be anything. Once, when my mother visited me at college, she learned that a housemate of mine came from Virginia. A moment after meeting she asked, "So was your family slave owners?"

I think of intervening, but I don't, and my mother suggests that Brian and I take off for the afternoon. She says to us, "I think Tyler can hold down the fort." I start to say something, and then I don't. We haven't had a real date since Porter was born and I'm curious to see the Mayan ruin in the jungle.

"If we time it to leave right after I nurse him, I think it might work for a few hours."

"It'll be fine—go," my mother responds. Both children are on her lap. All three of them smile at me.

After I nurse Porter, he is tired so I carry him against my chest to the beach and hand him to my mother. He nestles his head into the hollow of her neck and slides his finger back and forth against her cheek. He does this, strokes you with his fingertips when you hold him in your arms. Brian pulls on a T-shirt and I hand my mother a bottle just in case, and we climb into a VW bug that reminds me of the car in the movie *Sleeper*.

"It's strange to be alone," I say.

"It's *great* to be alone," he counters.

I reach for my seat belt, realize there isn't one, and grip Brian's hand. The road is one lane, potholed, and narrowed by a towering hedge on either side. The speed limit is the honor system. I involuntarily slam my foot on the floor when Brian says, "Whoa!" as a truck reels past and just misses us. Brian is unfazed.

I know we have made it when I see a stone pyramid poking over the hill ahead of us. We park in a sandy lot below an overgrown ruin and when we reach the base we find stone steps that lead up the back.

"I'll race you to the top," Brian says. "I prefer to compete with just-pregnant women." I take off running up the stairs and Brian lets me beat him.

"You're slipping," I say at the top. He stands beside me, barely huffing, like it was the easiest thing in the world. He was a nationally ranked wrestler and could still pass for one. When we compare arms, I look like the kid that the coach pushed into music class.

"Can you take a picture of us?" Brian asks a man. He nods, and we sit on a crumbly wall, smiling.

I start to get up and Brian pulls me onto his lap. "So what was that comment your mother made about Porter being secure?"

"You mean they didn't talk about attachment theory when you grew up in South Dakota?" I tease.

"No, we just discovered Romaine lettuce a few years ago. We never had that fancy tofu you got growing up either."

"I loved that stuff—ate it all the time."

"That explains a lot."

I make a face and lean down and kiss him.

"Let's walk over to the other building," Brian says, studying a map and pointing to a blob of trees in the distance. I see only vegetation but follow him because Brian knows where he is going.

Now, home from the hospital two months later with everything in disarray, I try to remember if I had any sense of the trauma in store for us. I'd read of a woman who said she had a feeling about being in a car crash one morning while she pulled on her pants. She said it felt like ice water poured down her spine, bouncing off each knobby bone. I couldn't help wondering why she got in the car anyway, but they didn't mention that detail in the story. I wish I could say I had one of those feelings about what was about to happen to Porter, but I didn't.

My back was as warm and dry as ever.

2

Brian and I married eight months after we met. I had moved to Minnesota from New York City, to settle my life and to try living somewhere completely different. I knew at this point that I wanted to become a psychologist, and took a series of jobs working with troubled adolescents and people with retardation before beginning a drug-education program at the high school where Brian taught. One of the things that first attracted me to him was the way he was effective in his life. He emanated competence and organization. He didn't get rattled. He was also six feet tall with dark hair and blue eyes and would make heads turn.

I counseled at the high school and we had gotten into a fight over a conference room. I was drawn to his stubbornness, or at least the unswerving way he stuck to his goal. It symbolized a certain steadiness in my mind. My life approach was looser and based heavily on luck. I felt lucky in life. I *was* lucky.

My life lacked a certain stability that might be promising in the long run. I realized this when Brian and I started dating. I saw how well he had organized his life and grabbed onto it with both hands, hoping my life could be streamlined by proxy.

We became involved later that fall and kept our dating a secret at first, in an attempt to shield it from the glare of students and fellow teachers. We were so successful in this effort that it wasn't until we got married that our colleagues learned of our involvement.

We decided to marry on the spur of the moment, prompted by the decision I had to make about graduate school. I had been accepted at Harvard and planned to go, though Brian was unable to come with me because of the joint custody of his children from his previous marriage. As a result, we were forced to discuss our future as a couple. We decided to get married, and I opted to begin a graduate program at the University of Minnesota instead of heading east. The month before classes started, Brian and I ran off and eloped.

We were married in a civil ceremony and then flew to Europe to begin a two-week honeymoon. Our first destination was Rome. We had taken a train from Amsterdam to Italy and walked through the station dragging our bags behind us, past the man in the army coat, the American tourists, and the pigeons darting out of the way. Everyone was smoking and pressing against me too tightly and I kept my eye on Brian's back, trying not to lose him. A man pushed postcards in my face and said something in Italian.

"Brian, wait," I said loudly.

He stopped and turned; he held his hand out to me, then pulled it back to let the postcard man pass by, and then grabbed for me again. We made it outside to the curb, where people hustled past me and the cigarette smoke made the air seem thick. As we walked, Brian studied the tourist guide *Let's Go Europe*, opening it to the chapter on Rome and the section on lodging. We were newlyweds with only our bags and our tour book, without a place to stay.

An old man touched my arm and asked, "Pension?" I said yes, and we followed him down the block to a stone house where he unlocked a courtyard door and led us up the stairs. The middle of each step was worn and smooth, and I looked at them and the narrow walls and the tiny man ahead of me as I held Brian's hand.

He opened the room without a key and I saw floor-to-ceiling windows that streamed in light. I glanced through them to the windy roads below.

"Okay?" the old man asked. We nodded and he left.

We avoided lying down, afraid we'd go to sleep and wake up in the middle of the night because of the time change. Instead, we put on running shoes and left for a jog towards the Colosseum in the distance. We ran on and off the sidewalks, tiny cars gunning past. My eyes on Brian's back, we ran in silence. We passed the bread shop and the outside café and more American tourists.

We made it to the Colosseum and climbed the steps, still huffing from the run. As we came out, I took a wrong turn and ended up lost on a street that I'd never seen. When Brian finally found me, he was laughing.

"Lost?" he asked.

"I'm not lost," I said, "just figuring out where our hotel is in relation to this unfamiliar street."

"How is this going to work if you join the police force?" he asked, cocking an eyebrow. I had told Brian from the start that one of my dreams was to apply my psychology degree to law enforcement: first join the police department, then the FBI.

"I can just see you driving in your squad," he continued, "when the dispatcher comes on, 'One Adam Twelve. We have a multiple homicide in progress west of you on Broadway.' And you'll say back, 'Uh, sorry, is west right or left of here?'"

"Yeah, you didn't exactly lead very well," I said, "What happened to you?"

"I was blocked behind about eighty-five girls in knee socks walking to school, and when I finally got free you were gone." We were both laughing, light-headed newlyweds.

"Come on—let's find some water—I'm dying of thirst," I said. We walked the block back to our room and changed clothes before heading out for a snack. I didn't notice the tourists or pigeons or cigarette smoke this time.

A month after returning from Europe, I began my PhD in neuropsychology at the University of Minnesota. Scrapping our initial plans to wait until the end of school, I was pregnant with Tyler in my second year, and had Porter sixteen months after she was born. Almost miraculously, my best friend from college, Nina, also started a psychology doctoral program at the University of Minnesota at exactly the same time. We had been close friends since our first week at Wesleyan, when, after an initial period of hating each other, we discovered we were soul mates. Both of our mothers were therapists and our fathers were college professors, and we related to each other with easy shorthand right from the beginning. We lived on the same dormitory hall as freshmen and baked chocolate chip cookies in her toaster oven on nights we deemed too cold to walk to the cafeteria.

I had never met anyone like Nina before moving to Connecticut. Her family drank wine with their meals and cooked elaborate Italian dinners, and she had spent a summer alone in Nantucket before beginning college. She was smart and ambitious. She was different from the kids in my hometown; they usually drove tractors for fun.

I could see from the start that one of the things that first attracted me to her was that, despite how smart she was, she had a tendency to just wing it. Nina also understood how tricky it was, and is, for me living with my brain, that there are things missing. She knows that I am spacey and have a tendency to lose my keys, but never judged me for it.

Along these lines, she is the only other person I know besides me who has driven through the front window of a convenience store while completely sober. She wasn't surprised, though she was quite sympathetic.

It happened like this: I pulled up to the store on a quick errand to get some eggs and I accidentally hit the accelerator, thinking that it was the brake. I know—it could happen to anyone. I was having what my father calls one of my "out-of-body experiences," in which I get just a tiny bit caught up in what I am thinking and tune out my immediate environment.

In a car crash, that thing you always hear about—time slowing down—really happens. I watch the car move forward towards the plate-glass front window. I hear the scrape of metal and wonder if I'll go through the wall. I go through the wall and see the candy display and things fly in the air. A muscle magazine lands on my window.

A pimply-faced teenager approaches my car, which sits on the brick base of the plate-glass window. The engine is smoking and this seems bad. He leans in the window and turns off the ignition. I sit there, stunned, and see a Twinkie package on my hood, then hear a siren and wait for the cops to come.

The cops appear. One is young and tall and runs the show. "I hit the wrong pedal," I tell him.

"That's helpful," he responds. I wonder what's happened to bedside manner. He leans closer to me, I hear a little sniff and I realize he is checking for alcohol. Satisfied there isn't any, he pulls his head back from the window and produces a camera.

"Are those crime scene photos?" I ask him.

"Nope, I just know my buddies at the station will want to see this," he starts laughing. "Can't say I've ever seen someone take out a convenience store completely sober."

I get out of the car on wobbly legs and the store clerk grabs my elbow like he's helping me cross the street. He is young, tall, and thin. If he were a painting he'd still have wet edges.

I see someone I know. The girl that lives across the street is staring. Her mouth is open and her eyes are big, she gawks at me without blinking. This seems rude, but maybe right at this moment I am not in a position to judge. I wonder if it's appropriate to crack a joke.

"Wow," she says when I get close enough to touch her. Her nails are painted black as if she's hit them with a hammer. I heard that she was caught smoking pot behind her parents' house and I feel the urge to turn the tables.

"Yeah, I had an accident," I tell her.

She looks at the front of the car resting against the candy rack. There is a ring of Snickers bars beside the left tire. The hazards are blinking.

"Makes me feel a lot better about the garbage can I hit last week," she says.

Nina understands these moments. There is something that calms me just being near her; maybe it's the lack of pretense, maybe the warmth, maybe the shorthand with a female friend that makes the quiet spaces comforting.

Nina and I lived together for much of college and sailed along, despite lost wallets and countless parking tickets. We weathered an ill-fated stint in the "Feminist House," our time there ended after Nina's boyfriend destroyed the front yard by doing wheelies in his Suburban. I moved out with her at the end of the year as a gesture of solidarity.

When graduate school began, we were back taking classes together, again wearing fashionable but inappropriate shoes in the snow, talking in psychobabble, and still baking cookies (though now we had graduated to a regular oven). Nina arrived in Minnesota shortly after I returned from my honeymoon, and even moved in with us for a few weeks when things were rocky with her Suburban-driving boyfriend.

When my children were born in the following years, Nina was there every step of the way and became a surrogate aunt and godmother to them. Nina understands me in a secret twin language. But even in our language there aren't verbs or nouns to describe what is happening to Porter.

With Brian and the kids to care for at home, my work and studies are my escape. It's my other love. My graduate school days were divided between classes and research. Each morning, I walked across campus over the underground bookstore, past Hillel House (where I ate kosher pizza) to the red brick buildings (always cold in the winter) for my psychology classes. My graduate research focused on two areas: working with dementia patients and studying people with Prader-Willi Syndrome (PWS), a rare genetic disorder.

My first introduction to the clients with PWS occurred when I visited a Minneapolis treatment facility called Birchwood in conjunction with a research study I was conducting. The center was located a few blocks from Lake Harriet and within walking distance to a quaint enclave called Linden Hills. Initially I'd never heard of PWS, even though it affected 1 in 12,000 babies. I learned that it was due to a genetic fluke that causes children to be shorter than normal and mildly mentally retarded (though their verbal skills are often exceptional). Most striking to me was the characteristic relentless focus on food. People with PWS ate two-pound bags of granulated sugar and entire roasted turkeys. They broke into their parents' padlocked refrigerators to eat sticks of butter and stole food from the corner convenience store. Before an effective treatment was found, they had always died young from weight-related problems—sometimes in their beds unable to move, sometimes in hospitals. Everything changed in the late 1980s when a group of Minnesota parents took matters into their own hands and created the nation's first treatment center for people with PWS.

At first glance, the treatment model seemed harsh—food was kept padlocked and clients were vigilantly supervised. The pantry window was broken twice on my watch, once with a rock and once with a fist. The residents were put on strict diets and forced to exercise regularly. They were weighed daily to ensure they weren't gaining any weight from stolen ketchup packets. I was drawn to these people and their utter inability to control an obsession with food.

My research consisted of measuring how far people with PWS would ride a stationary bike for a variety of snacks (the answer: until the tires blew out). The clients were quirky and charming and when my research officially ended, I signed on to be a counselor at the treatment facility because it was impossible to leave them—they warmed their way into my heart quickly. There was something straightforward and unmeasured in their approach to life that I admired. Typical workdays consisted of supervising meals (everything served with measuring cups), helping with daily routines, and conditioning the clients to stop swearing.

I finally understood the power of the eating disorder one Friday night when I worked the late shift and one of the residents suffered a psychotic episode. Such mental illness often coexisted with PWS patients, though was not caused by it. Barry walked past the staff office wearing a plastic garbage bag held up by his Graceland belt. Tipping his head into the doorway, he said to me sweetly, "I'm certain the rock era will end this century."

"Why are you wearing the Glad bag, Barry?" I called after him, but he was already gone. I jogged to his bedroom, where I found him talking loudly to himself, and realized that he was hallucinating. A second counselor and I brought him to Hennepin County Medical Center to get a psychiatric evaluation.

As we sat in the crowded waiting room next to barefoot children building LEGO towers, his symptoms grew worse. Eventually, he deteriorated to the point that he was lying on a gurney singing songs from *The Sound of Music* at the top of his lungs. Between each verse, he snorted like a pig.

As we waited for our turn, a young male orderly in high-top sneakers came up to move Barry to a quieter location. He asked, "How's he doing?"

Barry belted out, "How do you solve a problem like Maria?" Oink, oink.

The man took a step back, trying to look casual. "Would you like a sandwich?" Barry was still crooning, and I wasn't sure if he heard the question.

But then he sat straighter and sang, "So long, farewell, *auf Wiedersehen*, goodbye." He paused for a moment and I waited for the snort, but he added instead, "Turkey on white, please."

I loved being at Birchwood, listening to the residents fight over George Bush and hearing the *click-click-click* of someone testing the refrigerator's lock. I became immersed in their world. This was never clearer to me as when I found myself sucked into a fight over Diet Pepsi versus Diet Coke.

I voted for Diet Pepsi.

A week after Porter's seizure and hospitalization, I return to Birchwood and our lives slip back into a familiar routine. Everything is going to be all right.

In the late afternoons I pick up the kids and take them home to nurse Porter while Tyler practices the letters of the alphabet. We say "ga-ga G" and "huh-huh H" and Tyler beams when she gets them right, which is most of the time. After dinner, we move to the living room where we three lie on the floor and watch Porter as he tries to roll over. He gets one leg up and across his chest and is stuck like that. Sometimes I give him a nudge and he flops over onto his stomach.

When Brian goes back to work, Nina comes to visit. She is carrying magazines, chocolate, and toys, and I see a Starbucks bag under her arm. She makes a pot of strong coffee, then sits on the floor of my living room, playing with Tyler as we both sip our drinks out of giant yellow mugs.

She looks at Porter lying on the floor next to me. "He seems great, Sar, I can't even tell something happened." I nod my head because her comment makes me feel good. I nod to say that I agree, and everything is fine, even though I'm not positive I believe it. Nina looks at Tyler and says, "I was hoping you could come to my house to help me bake brownies."

"You don't have to do that," I say. I know that Nina is inviting her to give me some time with Porter. She knows that I need it, but I have trouble saying yes.

"It's not for Tyler," Nina continues. "It's for me. I just needed a good excuse to bake." Nina and Tyler head to her house for the afternoon and I hold Porter across my lap and nurse him. He drinks for a minute, then leans away and smiles. I say, "Keep going," but he just grins and purses his lips like he is blowing me a kiss. "You're not done yet," I say, and he leans his head towards mine and coos. We do that for a long time. I talk, he coos. I talk, he coos. Finally, he finishes nursing and falls asleep against my chest and there is a trail of milk dripping down his cheek. I scoot him over and lie down with him to take a nap on the couch. He never stirs. This is another thing that I love about Porter, how calm and easy he is to take care of. He loves to be held and starts smiling when he spots me walking into a room. I shut my eyes and stroke his head, then drift off to sleep myself. I wake up when I hear the back door slam, and then Tyler appears, smiles at me, and I can see chocolate around her mouth.

Later that afternoon, when Brian is home, we have dinner and baths and stories. We repeat this scene every night and as each day passes our lives feel more and more normal. Porter seems fine, and I tell everyone who asks about him how lucky we are. We will always be together.

Then two weeks later, he stops breathing. Just like that.

3

5 MONTHS

I am home alone getting ready for work and drying my hair as Porter lies beside me on a blanket. When I smile down at him, Porter's eyes are frozen and his lips are blue. I scream and put my cheek against his mouth to check if he is breathing. He is not. I don't feel anything. He's dead.

I grab the phone and punch in 9-1-1, tapping my foot through two slow rings.

"Emergency, can I help you?" the operator asks.

"My baby stopped breathing."

"Tell me what he looks like."

"His face is blue!" I scream, as I clutch Porter in my arms.

She says loudly, "You need to stop yelling so I can help you." I force myself to concentrate as she guides me through baby CPR, and I do the two-fingered presses until I hear the rescue truck pull up outside. We live a block away from the station so the firefighters come first, tromping up the stairs in blue coveralls and boots. A medical case like a tackle box bangs the wall beside me as they circle around Porter and then move me out of the way. A man drops to his knees and takes over for me until Porter starts breathing, one quick little gasp.

We scramble into the ambulance and the paramedic tucks a bear onto the stretcher beside Porter, saying, "The church ladies make these." I watch the numbers on the oxygen gauge flash every few seconds, holding my breath, fixated on the monitor.

Porter breathes normally on the ambulance ride over. I watch the gauge so I am positive about this, and he breathes all the way. I call Brian from the ambulance, only able to say, "Porter stopped breathing—he was blue, Brian. We'll be at Minneapolis Children's Hospital." We pull up to the emergency room entrance where a woman greets us by the automatic doors. She's holding a huge stack of files, signaling for us to hurry up with her one free hand. You didn't need to be an expert on body language to understand that she'd be calling the shots. She probably knew in kindergarten that she was going to be the head nurse.

I jog after the gurney as they wheel Porter into an examining room. I stand by the medical shelves filled with rubber gloves and plastic tubing. A doctor leans over Porter and looks at him, then listens to him and touches his face and I want to know what the doctor is checking.

Brian arrives, panting and pale, and asks, "How is he?"

Porter's face was cold.

"Okay," I say, "just sleeping, I think."

"What happened?"

Blue lips.

"It happened again." Brian puts an arm around me, but I don't want to be touched and I move away. We watch the people buzz past the table as Porter lies silently on his side.

"The seizure wasn't a fluke," Brian says after a few minutes, which is exactly what I am thinking and trying not to say. A doctor confirms this moments later, telling us that the vaccine can now be linked to an ongoing-seizure disorder, and Porter stopped breathing, as people sometimes do, in the middle of an intense episode. The doctor pulls a pad out of his pocket and jots something down with a tiny pencil that fits in the palm of his hand.

"I filed a report with the Centers for Disease Control about Porter's reaction to the shot," he says. "Do you know about the National Vaccine Injury Act?" I shake my head. "It's a program set up by Congress to compensate for the medical needs of children injured by vaccines. I think you might want to look into it." With that, he hands me a phone number and turns down the hall to answer a page. I tuck the paper into my pocket, reassuring myself that it isn't that bad. After all, they said that Porter just has epilepsy and it is very treatable.

Porter is wheeled into the Intensive Care Unit (ICU) for observation. Someone has to get Tyler from day care. "I want to be here to nurse Porter when he wakes up," I say, even though we were told Porter probably would not wake up soon because of the seizure and the multiple sedatives.

Brian pulls his coat on and says over a shoulder, "I don't feel right leaving, even though I can't do anything here."

"I need to stay here."

"Okay—that's fine. I'll be quick." He leaves and I'm alone. I stand by Porter's bed and stare so hard that little black dots fill my vision. I'm holding his tiny fingers when I hear Tyler's voice in the hall.

"Is he better yet?" she asks.

"A little bit. No more seizures."

We step out of the room as a nurse begins taking Porter's pulse. We go down the hall past the open area where the preemies sleep in glass boxes. I peer into the one closest to me and see a tiny baby with its eyes taped shut. The intensive care unit is bright and open to allow the doctors to move quickly around it. I try not to stare at the other children because I'm afraid I'll be overwhelmed. *Porter doesn't belong here*, I think, wedged between the crack baby and the girl born missing half of her brain. But at least he won't be staying long, the doctor said that once we had him stabilized on medication and the seizures under control, we'd be on our way once again.

Brian, Tyler, and I sit in Porter's room until 9:00 p.m. watching him, though he is unconscious. Tyler is getting squirrelly. It's time for her to go to bed. I tell this to Brian, letting him know he should take her home.

"Can I sleep in his bed with him?" she asks.

"No, sweetie, they need to be able to reach him easily."

"I wish I could stay, too," Brian adds.

"I think I should be here in case he wakes up so I can nurse."

"I hate having none of our family members in this state," he says. "I'll put the phone by the bed. Call me if anything changes—I can always bring Tyler with me."

"I will. Hopefully it will be a very quiet night."

"We'll talk in the morning." Brian scoops up Tyler and kisses my cheek. I watch them disappear from sight, wishing I could climb into the bed with Porter too.

Instead, I wake up in the middle of the night and open my eyes to total darkness.

For a minute I can't remember where I am—in California, Minnesota? Then it comes back in a flood and I hold my breath. I have a fleeting hope that it has just been a dream, until my arm swings out and hits the metal bar at the edge of Porter's hospital crib. I had been dreaming that I left a baby out on a balcony and the snow had fallen, entirely covering its body. Its skin was cold. The baby was dead. I know because its lips were blue.

Like Porter's.

I roll onto my back, wide-awake now, knowing I won't be going back to sleep. A picture of the dead baby keeps floating into my mind. I lie in the dark, listening to hospital sounds, feeling very small and alone. I wish my parents were closer. I want my father to explain to me what's happening to Porter. Growing up, he was my ballast. My father always knew what to do. He was steady and kind, even in very low moments—like when we had the marijuana incident in high school.

My parents had been out of town on vacation and I had made pot brownies with a group of high school friends. For reasons that made sense at the time, though I can't explain now, I decided to save the extra one in the freezer. It stayed there until the afternoon that I came home from school and Dad called me into his office to have a "talk." My father was always around when we rolled in after school since he was a writer and worked from a home office. He'd sit at the dining table with me as I did homework and encouraged me as I wrote my first stories. I have the stilted, painful first pages to prove it. My earliest memory of writing together was when he taught me about haikus as we traveled by train through Canada. He'd write the first line and I'd do the next one.

That day after school he had a funny look on his face and I walked down the hall to his office behind him. Papers were strewn around his desk and the light on the coffee table glowed.

I knew I was on thin ice when he began the conversation by saying, "Was there anything unusual about that brownie in the back of the refrigerator?"

I froze. Dad studied me with an earnest look before he steamed on. "Because I ate it and then got on the phone for a live radio interview. I found after a few minutes that I was having trouble following the host's point. But the worst part was the laughing. I finally had to get off the call when I couldn't stop the hysterical snorting."

A minute later we both started laughing, and then snorting, before Dad composed himself and raised an eyebrow. "That wasn't your best move."

"I know, Dad. I'm really sorry," I said. I was. He put an arm around me and gave me a little squeeze.

"I think the man I was talking to thinks I'm psychotic." Dad laughed. "It's okay. He doesn't make much sense even when I'm sober."

These memories course through my head and I miss my parents. I roll over on the hospital cot—lonely in the darkness—wishing my father were here, wishing I could hear my mother's voice. I have no idea what to do. Growing up with two humanistic psychologist parents, I'd come to believe that the world was a friendly place when you came right down to it. Even when difficult things happened they could be dealt with—it was just a matter of trying hard enough. I focus on this as I lie in the dark, the scent of Porter's baby blanket, which is balled under one of his arms, filling the air. I'll figure out a way to make him better; he'll be one of the success stories that makes other people want to hang in there and try harder.

I'll make him better.

It's 3:00 in the morning. I drink two Diet Pepsis and then lie in bed, twisting and turning. The night nurse pokes her head into the room and we smile at each other before she turns on a light and takes Porter's vital signs. I want to talk to her so I won't feel so lonely, but I can't think of what to say and she leaves. After she goes, I pull Porter carefully into my bed to nurse him and he falls asleep that way in the single bed beside me. I stay awake feeling him breathe, his tiny leg pressed against me, as I look out the fourth floor window as the people below me begin to rise for the day.

Taking any of the mainstream anticonvulsants is the solution for 85 percent of people experiencing seizures. Whether they try phenobarbital or Depakote or Mysoline, almost everyone has their problem solved. For those patients who are not cured by one drug, a second medication is typically added and this mix does the trick. I learn these facts when we meet with Porter's new pediatric neurologist, Dr. Garrison. He happens to be on call and comes to see us early the next morning before his clinic. He is young and optimistic.

He tells us there is a 98 percent chance that everything will be fine once Porter takes one or two medications for a period of time. Dr. Garrison is a good doctor who always explains things to us. "Unfortunately there are 2 percent of people that fall in the intractable category," he says. He has to tell me the facts. These are sad people. I imagine them in their helmets at soccer practice. I put this out of my mind. It almost never happens.

They'd started Porter on the anti-seizure medication phenobarbital while he was still in the emergency room and I cringe at the thought of giving my five-month-old a barbiturate. My graduate school reading on the topic suggests that it could impair a child's intelligence. I have bad associations with phenobarbital—my baby will take the drug that starlets abused in the book *Valley of the Dolls*.

I speak to the neurologist and he tries to placate me. "*The New England Journal of Medicine* just did a big study on the drug and found that it may lower IQ by five points," he says. "I don't think that small of a drop is even noticeable. In fact, the bigger problem is sedation, so don't be alarmed if he's very tired."

When Porter awakes the next morning, we begin the medication immediately. I mix the crushed pills into baby food and try not to think about it. I feed the mixture to Porter, then wait for him to go to sleep. After two hours of Porter's inconsolable crying, I am sure I'd misheard the doctor about the drug's sedating effects. When the screaming surpasses eight hours, an intern gives us a new diagnosis: "paradoxical agitation." For some reason a minority of children can become severely irritable on the medication and Porter turns out to be one of them.

It is the teenage girl in the pink smock that suggests a stroller ride, and it works perfectly as long as I never stop moving. At 11:00 p.m., the third shift nurses arrive and one of them tells me, "It would be best if you let him rest in his crib."

I stop to explain the situation while Porter screams at the top of his lungs, hitting the side of the stroller and turning bright red. "He's been crying ever since he started the phenobarbital," I explain, rocking the stroller back and forth.

"Have you tried nursing him?" she asks calmly, and I wish I could be calm too, but the stroller is banging against my thigh and I'm extremely irritable.

"He won't."

"We have an electric pump you can borrow," she offers.

"I'm off those," I say, remembering the only time I'd tried one and the suction cup got stuck on a nipple for more than ten minutes.

"Sometimes laying him on his back helps," she continues.

"We've tried on his back, his stomach, my lap, nursing, patting, and ignoring him—nothing works. Can you give him something to help him sleep?" I ask.

"No, we wouldn't want to give him another sedative. The phenobarbital makes them very drowsy."

I do another loop around the ward with the stroller, Porter screeching as we pass the nurses' desk in the middle with each lap. One of the nurses cups the phone closer to her ear because she can't hear a thing over all the yelling. Porter finally sleeps for a few minutes as we walk and I try to gently park it next to his crib, thinking that will be close enough. The minute the movement stops, Porter's eyes snap open and he begins to scream again.

Circling around the nurses' desk finally does work. At one point I hear the woman I'd spoken to earlier on the phone with the doctor. "We need to give him something—no one can stand the screaming anymore." At 1:30 a.m., Porter receives a sedative and I sleep until the start of *The Today Show*. This time I learn how to make sherbet.

Porter wakes up at 4:00 in the afternoon. With Brian teaching and Tyler at school, I am left to fill my time in the rocking chair beside his bed. After a few hours I can't take it; I feel antsy and worried and in need of adult conversation. I head for the parents' lounge to rummage through the refrigerator and watch *Oprah*. I wonder if the other mother has brought a horse in yet to nuzzle her comatose daughter. The lounge is empty and I take a seat on the vinyl couch. I glance at the television hanging from the ceiling as it plays a deodorant commercial. I listen to the woman talk about how confident she feels with dry armpits and I wonder how it could be that I am sitting here.

With Brian and Tyler gone, I am scared. I feel the kind of anxiety that makes my legs twitch. I have always felt connected to a large extended family and now, more than ever, I yearn to be back in California living near them. My loneliness makes me wish that I were a kid again, surrounded by the people I grew up with.

When I was eight years old, my parents joined five other families, buying ninety acres in Northern California, in a tiny town called Forestville, on which we built houses and a community center. The adults were a group of psychologists who met in the 1960s doing low-cost counseling in Berkeley. Living in the country, we farmed chickens, sheep, apples, and walnuts. Twice a week, all the families ate dinner together at the community center and every Saturday morning we worked on the property. We pressed cider, debated nuclear proliferation, grew marijuana plants, and heated our water with solar panels. I never noticed until later that I missed learning a few practical details growing up—like the fact that hot is always on the left of the faucet or that even-number highways go east-west and odd-number ones go north-south, no matter where you are in the country.

The adults weren't all hung up on traditional child rearing.

On Saturdays we met at the community center at 8:00 a.m. and worked on the property together until lunch. We discussed the day's jobs. After our "work day," we met at the community center for a potluck, followed by a volleyball game on the sandy court near the creek.

Our commune celebrated holidays and anniversaries as a group, and each of us children had a Coming of Age ceremony when we turned thirteen. The weekend-long event marked our transition from childhood to adulthood. On my thirteenth birthday, I began my celebration Friday night, meeting alone with all of the women in the group.

"You can ask anything you want to know about sex, marriage, love, or womanhood," my mother spoke for everyone and I asked my questions, and they answered all of them. It was no-nonsense, but informative.

"Why would you want to have sex if you aren't in love?" I didn't understand casual sex.

"Because it feels very good," one of the women named Fran said, "and you begin to develop more and more sexual urges as you get older. I can tell you though, it is much more wonderful when you love someone." Fran was trained as a physician so I figured she had to know what she was talking about.

"What is it like to be married to someone?" I asked.

"It's a wonderful friendship and a lot of hard work," Lyn said from my other side. "It is the best, deepest, and most interesting relationship you can imagine, but there are times you feel like you want to pull your hair out."

We continued talking until almost midnight, laughing and telling stories, passing bowls of mixed nuts and sipping on spicy hot cider. When it was time to go home, we hugged each other good night in the dark, and I walked with my mother down the twisty road past the creek to our house. The following morning, the entire community met for a ceremony in which I chose a second mother, Lyn, as she was someone that I felt particularly close to. Lyn was part-mentor, part-parent, and someone I deeply admired.

Now, being in the hospital with Porter, I long for those past years, maybe because of the good memories, maybe because the commune's adults took care of things for me. Sitting in the ICU, a parent myself, I feel adrift and unsure and wish I could go backwards, just for a little while, to start things over again, and avoid anything bad happening to Porter.

I think of Lyn. Having a second woman to confide in buffered things; it gave me a bridge from here to there, since my own mother leaned on me for support and we rarely budged out of these roles. As a child I was my mother's protector. I'd figured that much out since day one. I was the one who noticed the way she laid on her bed with the lights out on sunny days. I saw it and kept track of it all. Someone had to.

My mother would tell me things, too, when I found her all alone in the dark. She would pat the bed beside her and say that she wanted to talk.

I remember being eight years old. I ran into the house to change into play clothes. All the other kids on the block were playing a game of Kick the Can and I wanted to get outside and join them. I ran to my bedroom to put on shorts and saw that my mother's door was closed; I couldn't just leave her like that. I pulled off my pants from school and left them in a ball on the floor. I yanked on my shorts, the cutoff jean ones I made myself with a pair of scissors. I ran down the hall to her room to tell her that I was going outside.

My mother looked up when I came in. "Hi honey," she said in a tired voice.

"Hi."

She patted the bed next to her for me to sit down. I didn't know what to do. I could hear one of the kids counting outside, "Two, three, four, five," as he got ready to start the game. I could barely stand to be missing it. But I crawled over next to her and sat on the bed just half way. That way she would know I was only staying for a minute.

"I'm so glad you came in. I wanted to talk to you," she said. I bounced a little bit on the bed. I could hear my next-door-neighbor, Shannon, yelling something. Shannon and I both liked the same boy, Kurt, who lived in the corner house with the plastic flamingoes in the front yard. His mother had gotten the birds in Florida and said that they were classy. Once, Kurt had invited me inside and his mother had given us cream cheese and jelly sandwiches with the crusts cut off.

"I can talk for a minute," I told her.

"Okay honey." She let out a loud breath and lay back down, her cheek squishing into the top part of her arm.

I looked out the window, then sat back down. "I don't care about playing that much."

My mother spoke as if she were talking to herself. "My father abused me when I was your age and it left scars. I can tell you see this. You are very sensitive."

I nodded and held her hand.

"I still can hear his voice in my head telling me I'm worthless. It hurts. I know you understand this. We have a very special bond. You understand everything I am feeling." She was silent for a long time.

"I don't know what I'd do without you," she said. "I just get so tired sometimes. You're the only one who notices. It hasn't been easy."

"It'll be all right, Mommy." I felt like I was the only one she could count on when she said things like that. I felt like I could help her if I had the right books.

"I know, honey. Why don't you go play—I'll be fine. I'm just going to lie here a little longer." She patted my hand and rolled over. I knew I was supposed to help, but I wasn't sure how.

I hoped my father could help me figure out the perfect recipe to make her stop being sad.

He didn't.

After my younger sister was born, my mother flopped into her bed and didn't get up for two weeks. I brought her a pan from the kitchen and put it on the floor below her and waited. My sister lay in her crib but mom wasn't interested in her, as she was too busy studying the ceiling. I brought some water and the magazine she liked from the bathroom, and then piled them all on her bedside table and waited. I put my hand in front of her mouth to be sure she was breathing. I felt the warm air. Then I nudged her. When that didn't work I went back to my room and made a card for her—I drew a heart and wrote GET WELL SOON! on the bottom in fancy letters. It must have been a bad flu because nothing worked and she stayed like that until my father intervened and got her some help. In the meantime, we tiptoed and didn't make demands since she couldn't do it—any of it, end of discussion.

The helpless feeling I had with her, as a child, is the one I feel now, but it's different this time since I am the mother. I won't flop into bed. I won't give in. As I sit in the hospital lounge and stare out the window, I contemplate calling Lyn, but I don't want to have to explain the things I don't understand. Instead, I stretch out on the couch and flip through the television channels until I find a soap opera I've never watched. I close my eyes and listen to the dialogue, wishing I were someone else. I've veered or been dragged off my path.

4

"Seizures really aren't dangerous to people," the doctor begins, during one of the early morning checkups. I smile as he talks because it seems like making friends with the medical people is a good idea. He smiles back and says, "But people do occasionally stop breathing during one. So we're going to train you in CPR and send you home with a breathing alarm."

I don't know whether to feel relieved or terrified as Brian and I head to the parents' lounge to learn rescue breathing. We walk past the day surgery waiting room and the people inside look bored; I find myself wondering if any of them have ever seen someone turn blue. We get to the lounge and have our lesson, at which time we learn that we'll have to hook Porter to the breathing alarm at night; this will monitor his breathing so that any breaks in respiration will be detected and we will be notified by an ear-splitting whistle. The teacher pushes a button and the machine screams. We both jump and she turns it back off. As the woman shows us how to use it, she adds, "You'll be put on a special list for the electric company. That way, after a power outage, you'll be one of the first houses restored."

Brian tries to smile. "Thanks," he says, but I don't say anything because there is no good response to a statement like that.

Brian and I end up in separate CPR classes, so I find myself in a room with two strangers: the teacher and another mother named Renee. She has a son in the room next to ours who had a near-miss SIDS episode and was revived, so now they need a respiration alarm too. We take our turns breathing into the plastic mouth of a doll with eyes that snap open and shut. After the lesson, Renee and I hang around to talk.

"They don't have any Kleenex here, have you noticed that?" she asks. "I think they don't want us to cry."

I look around and can't see any—the only thing on the table next to us is Xeroxed copies of the *Patients' Bill of Rights*. "That's true," I say, wondering why I hadn't noticed.

"I'm going to run to Target and get some tissue—lotion-filled Puffs, in fact. I'm going to put them in every room." We grin at each other.

"Good for you," I say, wishing I'd thought of something like that. Renee gives a little wave and heads down the hall for the parking lot. I wish Brian had heard what she said about crying. Here we were in the hospital a second time and still hadn't discussed how we feel about what is happening to Porter. It strikes me as I sit by the CPR doll that we probably should talk about it so we don't end up miles apart: one of us driving to Target for Puffs, while the other goes home to water the plants.

Days later, we run into a roadblock when we try to reinstate our children back into normal life. Apparently, the biggest risk seizures can cause is an "absence of respiration." This risk is terrifying and untenable to Porter's day care center, New Beginnings. In short, the day care isn't big on kids that stop breathing. They say it more nicely than that, but this is the gist.

When he had his last seizure he needed CPR again. When we left the hospital that time, they told us Porter needed to be hooked to a machine whenever he sleeps. He needs to wear his breathing alarm even during naps. This entails sticking little circles to his chest, the kind you see attached to patients in TV shows when their hearts are hit or miss.

Hollywood leaves out the part about how there are babies that need them. They also leave out that babies have a tendency to yank off the wires. And that the monitors have the tendency to have false alarms. The first night sets the tone, when the alarm blares within minutes of Porter's bedtime. Brian jumps up and runs, then screams to me that everything's fine, the way cops yell "*Clear!*" when they don't find a gun.

Brian is less animated the next time and finally says nothing, except a sigh, as he slides back in bed next to me. We do this each night, trading shifts to reset the monitor, often finding Porter sleeping with the electrodes gripped in his hand. Maybe it is our technique.

I call the rescue breathing hotline and the teacher reassures me that babies get used to the electrodes after a while and stop pulling them off.

"How soon?" I ask.

"It's hard to say," she tells me. "Just double stick them on with packing tape."

I try the tip and it works, and after no breathing problems for weeks, I bring him back to his day care. I show her the electrodes and meticulously walk through how to turn the contraption off. I intersperse the whole thing with what I hope are witty comments about being on the power company's top ten users list.

The day care teacher looks nervous. She gets the day care manager who is adamant: They can't assume liability for babies that might die.

She does the dirty work and pulls me aside. She wears a sweatshirt that reads, "Cowgirl Up or Go Sit in the Truck." I want to cowgirl up, but I'm sent to the truck. "It's in our bylaws," the manager says, smiling. This means no but it's said in a nice way because she is a nice person, but no means no and Porter can't stay.

"It has never gone off with a real problem. All that blaring is false alarms," I say. I'm back in defensive mode. I hear it in my voice as if I'm listening to someone else. It is a person that I don't like.

"Our bylaws are very specific," she says. "Breathing is a requirement." She smiles again. I nod to show her I think breathing is important too. "We like Porter. We like you. We just don't like it when bad things happen."

It's hard to argue with that one, so I collect my son and his monitor and we walk towards the car as he chews on the wires.

Without a place to take him, someone needs to stay home, so Brian and I sit across from each other in the living room, devising a plan. He will stay home the next day so I can take exams. I will stay home Friday.

"I can't keep missing work," he says.

"I can't just skip exams." We are in a standoff, as we've both spent so much time at the hospital and doctor's office, we are dropping the ball. It is impossible not to think about lost jobs, a failed education, and other responsibilities.

I am sure we can make it work but just not sure how.

On my day off I start looking through the *Star Tribune* in a section called, "In Home Day Cares." One ad catches my eye: loving Christian mother, TLC, nutritious food. This sounds promising. I call the Christian mother and her name is Mary. We talk about her day care and I tell her about my children. I talk about Tyler first because Tyler is easy to talk about. Porter is not easy to talk about. I stumble through my description of Porter's condition and wish there were *CliffsNotes* for this kind of conversation.

I explain that Porter has had two seizures and uses a breathing monitor and what that means. There is nothing, so I keep talking. I wait for her to cut in and she doesn't and I talk more and still there is nothing. My heart bangs in my chest. The banging makes it hard to think.

Finally she says, "God places people in all our lives for a reason. You should bring him over, seizures don't scare me."

The following morning I bring the kids over. She is a loving woman and she hugs me when I step into her home.

The house is cluttered with toys and the kitchen counters are filled with Costco containers of cereal and animal crackers. There is a cross over the front door and a picture of Jesus gazing down from above the dining room table. In one bedroom, she has four portable cribs set up, pressed into each corner. She is calm and warm and I want to stay on her couch for the rest of my life. It is less the things she says and more the way she makes me feel. Her acceptance of Porter, his seizures, and breathing monitor washes over me and settles the agitated places inside me. I feel like we are home.

On Monday I bring Porter's monitor and a list of phone numbers to Mary's house and she takes a magnet and puts them on her refrigerator. There are pictures of her children, dressed in Little League uniforms and posing with bats. There is a smiling boy and a girl and they are lined up from littlest to biggest. My list of doctors is on her refrigerator next to the latest photograph.

I also give Mary something Porter's new neurologist, Dr. Garrison, gave us. It is a typed letter that explains Porter's "status seizures," or the kind that will go on indefinitely without drugs and more drugs. The note has instructions for the amount of intravenous Valium and Ativan he should get and how quickly subsequent doses can be given. The doctor lists these drugs as well as phenobarbital, something they shoot directly into Porter's bloodstream if the shaking won't quit. I have copied the note and laminated it, and hand it to Mary in case of emergency. I know what's written by heart. I leave the information for Mary to have because we never know what will happen. No matter how often we've been through it, each seizure scares me.

With Porter situated at Mary's house, things feel more settled and we dive as fast as we can into work. I've kept my Saturday shift at Birchwood with the PWS patients to help our cash flow. Birchwood is a converted nunnery and it still feels like an industrial park. Every entrance is locked so that no one slips out after dark to zip to the Super America for Cheez-Its. I am used to this now, as I also am to doling out the vegetables in a ¾ measuring cup and counting the number of grapes each client gets. My negotiating skills are sharp.

I get to the living room and I see that it's chore time, which is the time slot before dinner during which the clients do their housecleaning. I can hear an argument in the other room.

"Give me the vacuum you fucker!" It's Randy's voice and then I hear something muffled. I walk over and see Fran yanking the hose out of Randy's hand.

"She won't give me a turn," he says.

Fran looks and rolls her eyes. "He didn't ask nicely," she says.

"Maybe if you had a kinder way to talk to people you'd get better results, Randy." I say. He looks at me and gives a little shrug like it's the most idiotic thing he's ever heard.

He waves his hands like he's greeting royalty. "*Please* give me the vacuum, you fucker!" he asks. Fran hands it over.

When Randy is done vacuuming I find him at the staff office door, looking for me. He is holding a flower—something he picked outside, probably on his walk to the library. He holds it out to me when I get close.

"You are very attrap-tive," he says. For a minute I am stumped, running through the hunting terms I know. He starts tapping his foot and singing.

"Hey good lookin' . . . what you got cookin'?" *Tap, tap, tap*, I hear, as he taps his foot in time with the tune.

"Did you need something, Randy?" I ask.

He stops singing. "I want to give you this flower as a token of my friendship."

"Thank you, Randy. That's really nice. I'll put it in water."

I am glad that we are back on good footing. I hear him whistling as he leaves.

A few minutes later I hear him again and this time he is talking with the other men in the group a few feet outside the doorway. "You better not make the moves on Sarah, because I've seen her husband and he's really huge," Greg says. All of the residents know Brian from a picnic we had last summer.

"I heard he was a wrestler in college," Billy adds.

"He can pin you in five seconds. I heard he killed someone," Greg tells the group.

"I just gave her a flower," Randy says.

"Smooth move," Billy replies.

"We're *mainly* friends," Randy protests.

"It's your funeral," Greg says back.

Silence.

Then Randy appears in the doorway again. "You know I wasn't making the moves on you when I gave you that flower," he tells me.

"I know. It was really nice of you."

"Tell Brian it wasn't romantic."

"For sure, Randy. Don't worry."

He pauses a minute. "Can you give that flower to Brian as a token of my friendship?"

I think of this again as I come home from my shift that night to check on Tyler and Porter. They are fine and it's 11:00 p.m. so I roll into bed with Brian. After midnight I am thinking of something else—of the comment that the emergency room doctor told me about Porter's second seizure. "Some kind of brain injury has clearly happened." I lie in the dark, wondering if this means that Porter will struggle with school. Academics were a central value to my family as I grew up. In my junior high yearbook, a friend wrote, "Hope you like Harvard or wherever you are going." Both my grandfathers had attended Harvard and my father was admitted at sixteen. In fact, it wasn't a matter of whether or not you'd go to college in our family, but in what you'd get a doctorate. So I started my PhD at twenty-six and took all the tests and published the research articles, but soon realized there was another way my competitiveness surfaced—I wanted to have very smart children. It never crossed my mind to challenge the importance of my kids being Trivial Pursuit champions.

Deep down I know that Brian will figure out what is happening with Porter. He always knows how to fix things. He turned an unfinished attic into a master bedroom and bath during the first year of our marriage. He rotates things in his mind and visualizes blueprints and maps. He doesn't realize that normal people can't do this. The first time I went to his house he gave me directions on the phone. This was also the first time we argued.

"You turn on Portland Avenue, then go south," he said.

"South?"

"Then you turn east on 58th Street."

"How do I know which way is east when I've never been there?" I asked, frustrated.

He's stumped.

I march on. "What happened to just saying turn left or right?"

Brian adds this useful tidbit: "If you aren't sure, check the direction of the sun."

"That's a joke, I'm guessing." He can't be serious.

"Just check if it is over your right shoulder or your left," he tells me. *He is definitely joking*, I think. But he is not joking, and

I set him straight. He also learns to give proper directions in the future.

The next day I decide to look for answers.

My advisor in graduate school just happens to be a neurologist. He also happened to be the advisor to Dr. Garrison when he attended the University of Minnesota for medical school. Dave runs the neurology clinic at the university and I conduct testing for his patients who suffer from dementia. He's based his career on studying neurological dysfunction and he is familiar with research showing that pertussis causes neurological complications in some people.

After I tell him about Porter's seizure and second hospitalization, I ask what he thinks.

"Oh my God, Sarah, it sounds like a classic reaction to the pertussis shot. I've read some articles on that."

This surprises me. "But the pediatrician said that it couldn't be related."

He looks at me. "Then someone is covering their ass."

It was a high moment for me not to have an explosive reaction to this news.

"It's been awhile since I read about this, but the research is there. The Institute of Medicine and the British counterpart both recently issued statements on this. Go to the medical library and start there," he says.

I spend the following Saturday and Sunday at the medical library, buried in the stacks. This is usually one of my favorite places to go. I love the smell of the books, the tiny study areas, and the dim corridors on the underground floors. I dig through the shelves. Within an hour I have a pile of medical journals and skim through the data.

I learn about the basics of the pertussis vaccine. The symptoms of whooping cough are generated by the pertussis toxin, and the body fights it off by creating antibodies to the illness. This immune response tackles the toxin and neutralizes it.

That seems fine but there's a catch. Unlike many of the other vaccines, the whole-cell pertussis vaccine contains an active virus, and the same toxin that generates an immune response can also lead to symptoms of the disease itself.

I pause as I read this. I have a vague recollection of this kind of risk from stories of people who occasionally develop polio from their vaccine.

Sitting cross-legged on the floor, I hold a medical journal in my lap. Down the hall two students are pressed together in a carrel. I hear them whispering about chemistry and snatches of their conversation drift across the room. They are studying for their classes and I am studying for my son, and at the moment I can't remember why I ever cared so much about coursework.

I think of Porter and of his seizures and the breathing monitor and I wonder if he will ever get better.

One of the students kisses her friend and they laugh. They are happy. Yet I am reading about brain infection. I feel lonely and I wish I didn't—I hunch over and keep reading.

The floor is hard and my legs are stiff and I don't move. *I want to understand everything known about this vaccine*, I think.

I read three studies in rapid succession.

First, the history of the illness. When the vaccine was introduced, it was hailed as a miracle. Before that, babies died. There are accounts of them coughing so hard that blood sprayed out of their mouths—thousands of them every year. Children coughed so hard they broke their ribs, and the hacking rattled their bodies until they vomited. Their faces turned blue as they struggled to breathe.

The introduction of the pertussis vaccine stopped the deadly epidemic and the shot did things the best doctors at the time couldn't—it protected the children and kept the mothers from burying their babies. The shot saved people.

And, the shot hurt people.

Very rarely. But these reactions were brutal. The stories trickled into the medical journals and it became apparent that the whole-cell virus was a wild card. There were stories from across America and abroad. They were reported in journals in different languages, but the stories were the same. The outcome was also identical: In rare occasions previously healthy children reacted to the immunization with encephalopathy (disease, injury, or neurological malfunctioning) that resulted in permanent brain damage. I skim the descriptions of these events and it's a summary of what Porter experienced.

It's just bad luck, I think. *We lost the lottery*. I understand statistics and I understand pharmaceutical side effects—any drug has occasional bad outcomes.

I consider heading home. It is both disturbing and comforting to read that there are clinical words for what happened to my son.

Then an article catches my eye. It traces the history of the vaccine from inception to the current time.

I read about the vaccine's development in Japan, America, England, and the Faroe Islands. Vaccine programs evolved over time.

While the pertussis vaccine showed immediate results, the rare and darker events emerged as mass immunization occurred. Some kids, for some reason, had "bad reactions," as healthy babies became disabled ones. It had to do with the virus itself and the way it could generate the infection. There was a work-around, though. It conveyed the same protection without the toxic side effects. Safer versions of the vaccine with purified and inactivated toxin were produced and patented, and immediately demonstrated the ability to do the job without the casualties. The first of these was produced in America.

We were just too early for the safer vaccine, I think.

I read on. I flip through the pages to see when the new drug was developed.

1937.

My eyes see the date, but my brain won't believe it. *I must have read that wrong.* I look back at the article. I read it again.

1937.

That can't be right.

1937.

I flip through the article maniacally and track references the way I do when I'm writing a literature review for a class.

The story goes something like this: While the safer acellular version was marketed by Lederle Laboratories from 1944 to 1948, they stopped production when the same company introduced the Tri-Immunol DTP that still contained the old whole-cell pertussis. They hung onto the old vaccine formula for several reasons—it avoided the need for additional field-testing since it had been around so long. It was also cheaper to make.[1]

Over the next several decades, a number of different, safer acellular vaccines were created and used, though ultimately withdrawn from the market due to the additional cost associated with testing and manufacturing. The other reason many drug companies hesitated to launch the safer drugs: It would increase the liability they faced by continuing to sell the whole-cell pertussis when they had drugs available without the dangerous side effects.

The reports of problems continued to emerge and in 1948, *Pediatrics* ran an article that highlighted the severe reactions some children experienced following the pertussis vaccine. The abstract stated,

> Inspection of the records from the Children's Hospital for the past ten years has disclosed fifteen instances in which children developed acute cerebral symptoms within a period of hours after the administration of pertussis vaccine. The

---

1 Randolph K. Byers and Frederic C. Moll, "Encephalopathies Following Prophylactic Pertussis Vaccine." *Pediatrics* 1, no. 4 (1948): 437–57.

> children varied between five and eighteen months in age and, in so far as it is possible to judge children of this age range, were developing normally according to histories supplied by their parents. None had had convulsions previously...[2]

All sorts of other clues were suggested as to why some children were so sickened while most were just fine. Certain things stood out: Most of the bad reactions occurred in males, and many of these boys had family members with "nervous system irregularities." One thing was clear: The vaccine caused encephalopathy, something they knew definitively when they found cell-related abnormalities in the spinal fluids of the sickest children.

The combination of these case reports piece the story together. The researchers suspected that the reactions resulted from a specific toxin or from an antigen-antibody response. I write down the conclusion of one of the first articles in *Pediatrics,* "The present study has left these etiologic considerations unanswered, but it has called attention to a risk of the prophylactic use of pertussis vaccine not hitherto recognized." The reactions were severe and the reactions were rare, but they stacked up over time and were reported in each country where the immunization was used. By 1972, six major pharmaceutical companies had developed the safer acellular version of the DPT, but all six scrapped plans to market them for decades due to cost and liability reasons.

Ultimately America's response was slower than government action elsewhere. Other countries moved more quickly to the acellular version of the immunization. In the 1970s, the Japanese government sent Dr. Yuji Sato to the National Institutes of Health to study alternate pertussis development. In a 1982 *Lancet* article, Dr. Sato reported that his acellular immunization

2 Byers and Moll, "Encephalopathies Following Prophylactic Pertussis Vaccine." 437–57.

conferred nearly 100 percent immunity while containing less than 4 percent of the active pertussis vaccine.[3] Additional studies in the early 1980s revealed that the Japanese acellular version was equally protective to its whole-cell cousin, but had a rate of 83 percent fewer complications. Similarly, in 1979, Sweden banned the use of whole-cell pertussis in vaccines because of the rare brain damage to previously healthy children.

In the United States, the same frightening reports emerged. In response, in 1984 Dr. Alan Hinman and Dr. Jeffrey Koplan at the Centers for Disease Control (CDC) created a simulated model of one million American children to evaluate the risk-benefit ratio for the pertussis vaccine. Their research concluded that the benefits of immunization outweighed the risk despite the fact that one out of every 1,750 children experienced seizures and shock after their vaccine; one in 110,000 children developed encephalitis; and one in 310,000 children would have permanent brain damage. Their numbers estimated the impact for each pertussis shot a child received, not accounting for the fact that properly immunized children are given several doses of the medication before they start kindergarten.[4]

I read the American government's response in the 1980s and then how the issue was handled in England. In response to parental outcry, the British government funded and launched the National Childhood Encephalopathy Study (NCES) as a prospective means for tracking the potential association between the whole-cell pertussis vaccine and neurological damage. The study reported a list of conclusions:

- Most of the country's cases of neurological dysfunction and disability were non-vaccine related.

3 Yuji Sato, Motoo Kimura, and H. Fukumi, "Development of a pertussis component vaccine in Japan." *Lancet* 1, no. 8369 (1984): 122–26.

4 Alan Hinman and Jeffrey Koplan, "Pertussis and Pertussis Vaccine." *Journal of the American Medical Association* 251, no. 23 (1984): 3109–113.

- Nonetheless, neurological illness occurred within a three-day window following immunization at a rate greater than chance.
- The prognosis was good for most of the children who experienced a bad reaction and the majority of them made a complete recovery in one year.
- Because of the increased rate of neurological illness following DTP, it was likely that permanent damage some children experienced that was caused by the vaccine was a "real but rare event."[5]
- The US government's response: In 1991 the Institute of Medicine (IOM) independently analyzed the NCES data and concluded that there was a rare but definitive relationship with encephalopathy in the immediate post-vaccination period, even though there was no definitive evidence that permanent brain damage occurred. The jury was still out, and more data was needed.[6]

Having conducted original research as part of my doctorate, I know the criticality of tracking the long-term impacts of the people studied. I scramble to find the longitudinal research on the kids who had a neurological reaction to the DTP. It strikes me that some interplay with genetics must be at work. Everything from fish to alcohol to nuts is tolerated by most people, and toxic to others. I imagine I'll find a well-controlled study examining the effect that whole-cell pertussis has on biodiversity. Nothing.

5 Alan Hinman and Jeffrey Koplan, "Pertussis and Pertussis Vaccine." *Journal of the American Medical Association* 251, no. 23 (1984): 3109–113.

6 Christopher P. Howson, Cynthia J. Howe, and Harvey V. Fineberg, *Adverse Effects of Pertussis and Rubella Vaccines: A Report of the Committee to Review the Adverse Consequences of Pertussis and Rubella Vaccines* (Washington, D.C.: National Academy Press, 1991).

Then it strikes me: I'll read through the follow-up conducted by the CDC on the children our vaccine court has acknowledged were brain damaged by pertussis. The programs started in 1986 and I search through the data to find long-term follow-up on these sure cases. Nothing.

I find that thousands of children have won their cases and thousands of children have their ongoing medical problems paid for by the National Vaccine Program. But aside from the statistic, there is no other information. Finally, I give up.

I leave the library. It is completely dark as I walk to the car. I went into the stacks for answers. Instead, my brain is packed with questions.

On the drive home my mind races. I think of how I signed the consent form when Porter received his pertussis vaccine. I knew rare complications could occur. I jotted my signature below a paragraph that explained these possibilities and I acknowledged they'd warned me that brain damage occasionally occurs. However, I didn't know when I signed that form that there was a different safer version of the drug. A version that other countries had used for decades and was proven to minimize these reactions. The United States finally replaced the whole-cell pertussis for mandated infant immunization. But, not until 1995.

I pull into the garage and Brian and the kids are in the living room. When I lie on the floor to relax, the phone rings. It is my mother. I move to the kitchen for the call and I relay all the latest facts to her. The exchange is a typical one that epitomizes something else about my mother: She's wired to save the underdog. This element of her is a result of the abuse she experienced. I know this since she spent hours when I was little telling me the fine points of her childhood torture. She's channeled this pain into adopting any rescue animal within fifty miles. Now she wants to go after whoever has hurt her grandson. I sit on a barstool in our kitchen listening to her.

"You need to sue the vaccine maker!" she says. She is revved up. My mother is often revved up. As we talk Tyler sits on the floor in front of me. She is reading a picture book and points at the page and laughs.

"How do you sue a drug company?" I ask. I can't imagine this. My mother can. She protested nukes in our years in the commune and once called the police because our neighbor was hosting cockfights. Then she found out the neighbor was the sheriff. Now she wants to go after Big Pharma. I listen to her tirade and don't say much. At the moment I am more concerned with whether the phenobarbital will make Porter flunk kindergarten. Or whether I will ever have sex with my husband again.

"I'm going to call Don!" my mother exclaims. She will get to the bottom of it. She always does. Don is an old friend and a lawyer, not the kind who sues drug companies, but the kind of lawyer who knows the kind who sues drug companies.

My mother runs through the game plan in a hurried voice.

I don't take it too seriously, to be honest. I am too busy cracking the code on seizures. The next morning I spend the early hours reading motivational books to egg me on. They are stacked on Porter's bedside table with enticing titles like *Self Help for the Bleak.* They say it is important to face the facts. I operate in reality technically, but focusing on the present moment isn't helpful.

My mother calls Don, who calls another lawyer. Then Don calls me. "I have a friend in a San Francisco firm who specializes in personal injury. He said he'd be happy to talk with you."

I write the number down on a pad with a smiley face. I sit down, still holding the pad, and impulsively dial the San Francisco lawyer's number. I'm told that he will call me back within the hour. I tap my foot while sitting at our kitchen counter. *Now we'll solve this,* I think. This is action. I love action. If I can't stop the seizures, at least I can hold someone responsible. That's what I think as I draw six more smiley faces on the pad next to the phone.

The lawyer calls and he seems like a nice man. This is good news. "I do personal injury, but you can't sue vaccine makers," he tells me. This is bad news.

"Why not?" I ask.

"They have immunity from liability." This strikes me as funny and I laugh in a manic way. I imagine he thinks Porter isn't the only one with problems.

"Immunity?" I say.

"Bad choice of words," he says. "The government has an arrangement with them that if they will make the vaccines they won't be held responsible for any side effects."

My wheels are turning. I'm revved up. *How do I take action if no one is responsible?*

"So that's it? What about those forms you sign that say you acknowledge the side effects that might happen?" I ask him, confused.

"They have a special court system for those that fall under the Vaccine Injury Compensation Program," he explains. My memory flashes back to the ER doctor the first night that Porter was hospitalized. He wrote the name of the program on a piece of paper and I had saved it in my sock drawer under Brian's love letters. I sent out for information, but never opened it when it arrived.

"Okay, so can you sue them in that program for us?"

"I don't do those kinds of cases," he says. I tap my foot. This is bad news. I draw a face with a frown over all the smileys.

"I know a woman in Minnesota that does handle those types of cases. Her name is Katherine Thompson and I can give you her number." I cross out the frown. I jot down what he says. I've never talked to a lawyer before in my life and now I have a third one to consult within two days.

I dig through my desk and find the documents that I received from the National Vaccine Injury Compensation Program (VICP). I read through them twice. I want to be prepared for our meeting with the lawyer. The documents are in a form letter style and explain that the 1986 National Childhood Vaccine Injury Act (Public Law 99–660) created something called the National Vaccine Injury Compensation Program (VICP). The opening paragraph is reassuring and clear. The primary purpose of the law was to balance public safety and the small risk that forced vaccination carries. It aimed to juggle the need for a consistent supply of vaccines while compensating the children injured or killed by their administration. The spirit of the act was to sidestep the traditional tort process for resolving vaccine injuries and create a process similar to no-fault auto insurance. In essence, someone does take the fault, though it is the US government instead of the pharmaceutical companies. Vaccines are the only products in America that are universally mandated for purchase by everyone in the country. At the same time, the manufacturers are exempt from liability.

"Table injuries," or those known as side effects of the various vaccines (found on an actual table), are agreed to be settled in an efficient way that provides compensation for the care of injured children. I can see why we might need help with the medical expenses—between the ambulance rides and ICU visits and medications and monitors, Porter's bills keep climbing and none of them are covered fully by insurance.

The vaccine court is a brick-and-mortar place with full-time judges overseen by the US Court of Federal Claims. These proceedings happen in a unique and separate court system run by "special masters." These are judges schooled in vaccine safety and injury who devote all of their time to handling these cases. I am excited to learn that the process is touted as humane and fast.

I sit with Brian at the dining table after the kids go to bed. I am excited and feeling extremely revved up. I have read all the documents and cut to the punch line. "These cases are settled fast! They are required to be done within 240 days. We can make it six months." I push the stack of papers over to Brian.

"It's hard to believe it will go that fast," he replies. We're playing our parts: I'm the enthusiastic but misguided motivational speaker and he is the calm and realistic counterpoint. His skepticism pushes my buttons just the tiniest bit.

"You're right, they will give a 150-day extension if it is a tricky case, but the whole point is to move you through fast so that they can help pay for the medical bills."

I launch into the background since Brian is thorough and analytical. He likes details. I hate details. By transitive property this could be a relationship problem, but as I think of the reconciliation needed on our medical bills and the records and receipts needed to file a claim, Brian's detailed style is nothing but an upside.

We sit side by side at the dining table and read through the documents together. "The compensation program is funded by a surcharge on the shots, not the drug companies," he tells me. In other words, our taxes pay for the care of the brain damaged children. The VICP is located in the US Department of Health and Human Services (HHS) and funded entirely by taxes on each inoculation. Every time a child receives a vaccine, a seventy-five cent charge is added. Multi-dose vaccines, like the measles, mumps, and rubella (MMR), add $2.25 to each administration, since the shot contains three separate vaccines. The collected money goes into a pool called the Vaccine Injury Compensation Trust Fund and is managed by the Treasury Department.

"It says they've paid over a billion out for the kids that are injured," I say, feeling relieved. I point to the official statement on the Fund, "The Vaccine Injury Compensation Trust Fund provides funding for the National Vaccine Injury Compensation Program to compensate vaccine-related injury or death claims for covered vaccines administered on or after October 1, 1988."[7]

"It seems too easy," Brian says.

"It is easy," I offer. My voice is determined. And loud. And bossy.

I shuffle around the papers to distract him. "The lawyer will tell us how to figure it out. It's her full-time job."

We drop the conversation.

The next morning we bundle up the kids and drive downtown after work to meet our potential lawyer, Katherine Thompson, an attorney in Minneapolis who represents families in the National Vaccine Court. A few weeks ago we had no idea this system existed, and now we are meeting with a lawyer who has worked full-time in this court for years.

---

7 "National Vaccine Injury Compensation Program." U.S. Department of Health and Human Services Health Resources and Services Administration. http://www.hrsa.gov/vaccinecompensation/index.html.

5

6 MONTHS

In Katherine's office there are pictures of her children on the desk and her law degree framed on the wall. She wears a business suit and has shoulder-length blonde hair. She looks like a cross between supermodel and class president. I think, *she can't be that polished*, but she can and she is.

She nods as we tell our story. I wait for her to cut in and to tell us vaccines are safe. She doesn't.

"It sounds like a classic case of encephalopathy caused by the pertussis vaccine."

"He was fine the morning before the shot and ahead of all his milestones before the first seizure," I say, still lobbing out my evidence. I want to add that we don't believe in conspiracy theories, and we aren't hysterical. But that sounds slightly defensive.

"Yes, that's how the cases go. Yours is open-and-shut," she tells us. I'm thrown off that she is agreeing with us.

"You've seen this before?" I ask.

"Yes, back in 1986 Congress passed the National Vaccine Injury Act to protect pharmaceuticals from liability and to compensate the kids that are injured or killed by vaccines. They hired medical experts to create a table of the side effects caused by various immunizations and what you describe is a severe reaction to the pertussis shot. It can cause a brain infection and brain damage. Seizures are a common part of that."

My eyes dart to Brian without turning my head. Katherine pulls a piece of paper out of a binder and shows us the table with reaction symptoms. They are listed in order of seriousness from slight to horrible. We are not at the bottom. That seems good. The bottom one is death.

I. Vaccines containing whole-cell pertussis bacteria, extracted or partial cell pertussis bacteria, or specific pertussis antigen(s) (e.g., DTP, DTaP, P, DTP-Hib)	A. Anaphylaxis or anaphylactic shock	4 hours
	B. Encephalopathy (or encephalitis)	72 hours
	C. Any acute complication or sequela (including death) of an illness, disability, injury, or condition referred to above which illness, disability, injury, or condition arose within the time period prescribed	72 hours

The table lists and explains injuries/conditions that are presumed to be caused by vaccines. It also lists time periods in which the first symptom of these injuries/conditions must occur after receiving the vaccine. If the first symptom of these injuries/conditions occurs within the listed time periods, it is presumed that the vaccine was the cause of the injury or condition unless another cause is found. For example, if you received the tetanus vaccines and had a severe allergic reaction (anaphylaxis) within four hours after receiving the vaccine, then it is presumed that the tetanus vaccine caused the injury if no other cause is found.[8]

"So we will sue them?" I ask. I am starting to sound like my mother.

"It's not suing, per se. We will file a claim in the court in Washington, DC. They have judges there called 'special masters' whose full-time job is to evaluate vaccine claims."

"Do you think we have much of a chance of winning?" Brian asks. I am thinking this but I don't ask. I love Brian's practical side—he gets right to the point.

"You have a straightforward case. I mean that. Records from the first night of the injury, the ER doctor noting it as a bad reaction, the report to the CDC of his severe reaction that night, and the subsequent problems. The court is set up for no-fault swift justice and it's feasible we'll have this settled in a few months," Katherine replies.

I feel elated. We will close the case and pick up the trail away from here.

Brian looks like he's solving a geometry equation. I can see he is already plotting logistics. If he were ever lost in the wilderness, he'd be one of those people who would survive for months with just their shoelaces and an army knife. I would have all of my pathologies triggered and be dead in two days.

He pulls a folder out and starts taking notes. "What are the steps?" he asks Katherine.

"The first threshold is met when you document that you've spent $1,000 out of pocket to cover expenses related to the reaction," she says. I give Brian a knowing look, and he raises his eyebrows back. The bills from the hospitalizations

---

8 "Vaccine Injury Table." U.S. Department of Health and Human Services Health Resources and Services Administration. http://www.hrsa.gov/vaccinecompensation/vaccinetable.html.

started arriving within a week of Porter's first stay. One for the ambulance, another for the time spent in the ICU, and separate ones for various doctors. The thousand-dollar mark was passed right out of the gate and we seem to receive new bills each week.

"They require the thousand-dollar threshold to be sure that nothing frivolous is filed. After you've hit that mark you need to collect all of his medical records showing what happened and we'll file them in the court," Katherine says. "They may ask for a few additional tests to rule out other causes, but it shouldn't be too difficult."

And just like that, our problem is solved.

Or just like that it seems our problem should be solved. The path is harder than we think. I see it immediately when the reality of gathering the data begins. It is slower and less inspiring than a trip to the Department of Motor Vehicles and my ability to speed the process is nonexistent.

I read through the guidelines for a ". . . prompt and efficient resolution of a claim." This sounds promising. I imagine we will tackle this case head on, but as I read the small print of a document from Katherine I have my doubts. Vaccine cases have two parts: first a verdict regarding the injury itself and then a damages phase in which the special master decides whether damages are warranted.

The first phase has an innocuous-sounding point that says parents' suspicions need to be firmly grounded to avoid giving the enterprise a bad name. Specifically, claims need a "completeness of records." This is straightforward enough, like crossing off the items on a preflight checklist. We need to file a "Rule 4," a document that encapsulates this data and spells out our legal arguments. This is not a black-and-white process because the special master decides if the evidence is complete. If not, he will order that additional expert input is needed.

The murky part turns out to be spotting the finish line. We turn in our documentation about the night Porter was injured, with the ER records and notes from the attending physician. The same doctor happened to be in the ER on our second trip there when Porter stopped breathing.

We hit a barrier when the government lawyers from the HHS push back and say that we haven't reached the evidentiary standard to prove Porter qualifies to file a claim. This happens in our very first status call with the judge. Katherine objects and they object and in the end the judge sides with the government and sends us back to the starting line. We are asked to go back to the lab, meet with another neurologist and a neuropsychologist, and get a detailed EEG reading to round up more facts. It dawns on me what Katherine means when she says we need to pace ourselves because the process is one that requires sneaking up on the truth versus tackling it all at once.

Despite my mixed feelings about Porter taking phenobarbital after his second long seizure, the drug works. This really just means Porter continues along in the following weeks without a blip. His body begins to acclimate to the drug and slowly he is in a calmer state. After a month on the drug he is languid but calm, and he has the dazed look of someone who's taken too many Benadryl. He starts to drool. We will eventually need to get him off the meds. Drooling is a problem in a job interview.

I think about this today as I spend the afternoon at Birchwood doing role-plays with Billy. We've named this exercise Personal Problem or Real Emergency.

I sit across from him in the tiny staff office and lay out the scenario. "You are on break at the Opportunity Workshop and you open your lunch bag and find that your sandwich is missing. Is this a real emergency or something you can handle on your own?"

Billy stands up and reaches for the phone over my shoulder. "An emergency—I'm going to get the police involved right away."

"Wait a minute—I think it is actually something you can handle with a counselor at work."

"You think so?" He is puzzled.

"I'm certain. Let's try another. You are home for a visit and you notice smoke blowing under your door. Is this an emergency?"

"Is someone barbequing?" he asks.

"No—but there is a lot of smoke and it seems very hot. What should you do?" I prod.

"Call Grandma?" he replies, with a note of doubt in his voice.

"No. This would be a good one for 9-1-1. You call the number and you get the police. What do you say?" I encourage him to continue.

"I'd tell them to get over here right away and arrest the sucker who stole my sandwich."

We decide to take a breather.

Billy is a new resident at the center; he was kicked out of his group home the week before. The facility was no match for the eating disorder. They quickly discovered this when he gained twelve pounds in the course of two days.

I talked with the program coordinator the day before Billy joined us and she explained the final straw. "He figured out how to take his screen off and climb out of his bedroom window at night. He grabbed a duffel bag and flashlight and made his way to the all-night Cub Foods down the road. Security was lax after midnight, and he managed to fill the bag with candy and hide it behind the house. We discovered a few days later that he was sneaking out after dark to consume dozens of Kit Kats in the woods."

In our facility the windows are thick Plexiglas and won't slide all the way open. So far, Billy has lost three of the twelve pounds he gained at the group home.

After our role-play, I sit with Billy and the other residents as they chat in the living room. They argue with unique perspectives on politics and war, religion and sports teams. They hash through their views on the afterlife, and Jerry tells the group about a recent vision he had.

"Listen," he says, "I know what I'm talking about—I've been to heaven and I've been to hell."

Billy perks up. "How was the food?"

We've moved out of the realm of having real emergencies in our lives. Another month passes without seizures and I'm pretty sure we are home free. In fact, things are so calm that we decide it is time to move into a new house.

It is only two miles away, but away from the flight path and closer to the park. Our dream of simplifying life has never gone away and we take a baby step towards this plan by moving into a simpler space. One Saturday we pull together a group of friends and carpool our belongings to the new place. Porter is thrilled by the crowd and wobbles around on hands and knees in the new living room, dragging a blanket behind him. He sits on the patio pouring water between two plastic cups while we eat pizza in the backyard. He does this for an hour. I realize this is a strange habit, but I like that it keeps him content.

Our first night in our new house, we have dinner and baths and stories as usual. Bedtime goes so well that I find myself stretched out on the couch, a fan blowing in my face as I read a back issue of *People*. This is the life.

Then things fall apart.

Porter wakes up screaming and won't go back to sleep. By half past two in the morning, I am insane, hating my new house and wondering how Brian and both kids have developed irritating traits simultaneously.

Finally, I've had enough for one night. I load Porter into the car and tell Brian I will drive him around until he falls asleep. I don't even think about an outfit for the ride. It is only when the flashing lights appear behind me and the officer walks up with a flashlight that I realize I'd been driving in a bra and underwear.

The cop knocks on the window. I roll it down.

"I had to drive around," I say to him, pointing behind me at Porter. "It was kind of an emergency."

He shines the flashlight over my shoulder to illuminate Porter's snoring form. "I'm sure it is," he says. Then he turns off the light and walks back to the cruiser.

Another month passes without a seizure, then two more weeks, and my confidence rises. I feel like a winner since we've stayed out of the hospital. We are normal and we do normal family things. Brian and I have a date night and we don't talk about seizures once. I think that perhaps I was overdoing it, that maybe Porter's issue isn't as bad as it seems. I go to work and the phone never rings telling me I need to rush back to the hospital. I talk about our problems in the past tense and feel a little embarrassed I thought we should file a claim.

I call Katherine to say that we are just fine. We've filed with the vaccine court, but it may be time to withdraw our petition.

"Still collect the records," she suggests.

She can be a buzzkill.

6

9 MONTHS

I think about why Porter's injury happened and what it means. My brain does this whether I like it or not, assuming there's always a way to squeeze some meaning out of difficult things that happen. I've always believed that any bad event singly is never the whole story anyway, since the world is a good place. With the connectedness of life, it is impossible to know what is really happening or why, at any given snapshot of time.

My go-to solution for most things is reading. One morning before the kids are awake, I find myself pulling a book by one of my favorite authors, Buckminster Fuller, off the bookshelf and a quote catches my eye. He believed in the interconnectedness of everything on Earth and the idea of precession or the endless chain of effect that all of us have on one another. It's similar to the Buddhist idea of dependent origination—that everything occurs as a result of a number of other factors and continually influences all of life around it.

Fuller believed that because no event is isolated, all of them have greater relevance. The trick is that the meaning is often hard to find in the moment. The significance may lie in the impact that the person or event has on everyone else. I catch my breath sitting cross-legged below my bookshelf thinking, *Something bigger is happening here. Nothing is a dead end. I will look back on what happened to my son and see all the ways it made us into stronger people.*

After breakfast the kids and I go outside. It is bright and we squint; the ground shimmers with the first snowfall.

The typical course of taking phenobarbital after a seizure is a year. Dr. Garrison said that after that stretch you can assume things have settled and most kids are never afflicted again. But things go so well—meaning Porter is not in an ambulance for three months—that we take him off the medications sooner. I push Dr. Garrison to taper him faster, since the sooner he's off, the sooner he's normal. Brian pushes too. And it works. We make up for lost time. We take both Porter and Tyler to the park and run them both around Lake Harriet in the baby jogger. It's sad to think about the people in the bad percentage the neurologist told us about, the ones that keep taking drugs and keep having seizures.

After the run, I take the kids to Rainbow grocery store to shop for dinner. I park the car and unload the kids, smiling at a man wearing a helmet who is wheeling carts. Since I am an insider, I know he has seizures. I say hello in a voice that is too chipper and he is surprised and stares at me. I give a little wave and lift Porter's baby seat into the cart. Tyler always drives.

I have my back turned when I hear the scream. It's the shriek of an animal as its leg is clamped into a metal trap. I've never heard the sound but I know that's it. Another scream. Poor animal. I whirl around and see Porter arching in his seat. His eyes roll up and they are white and his arms whap the side of the cart. I freeze. This isn't supposed to be happening. It's not supposed to happen so I can't move and only stare.

"Porter's having a seizure!" Tyler screams, and I reach slowly, unbuckling his seat belt and holding him on his side. His hands whap my arm and he groans with each lurch. Tiny bubbles seep from the corner of his mouth.

"He's having a seizure," I repeat. I rock from foot to foot because this isn't supposed to be happening.

A man in a green apron rushes over from the bakery. "Do you need help?" He knows I need it but still asks.

"Call 9-1-1," Tyler says.

"Call 9-1-1," I repeat. The man turns and runs behind the counter. He calls 9-1-1. People gather around in a semicircle, whispering. Tyler looks determined and I can't read the expression on her face.

I am sitting on the floor with Porter on my lap. His arms twitch. There is more foam at the corner of his mouth. The semicircle of people is ten feet back. No one comes close. Seizures keep people at a distance. Tyler sits beside me and pats my back. I am oddly calm, as if this is happening to someone else. I should be comforting her, but I am watching the scene and it unfolds without my direction.

I hear the sirens. The firemen come first and one gets on the floor next to me and talks into a radio. The knees of his pants are scuffed like a kid's. I wonder if he ripped them by kneeling down to resuscitate people.

"Has he ever had a seizure before?" he asks and I tell him yes, he has, and that they stopped and weren't supposed to start up again. He puts Porter on his side until the paramedics arrive and Porter is strapped onto a stretcher, then loaded into the ambulance. Tyler and I join them. His arm hits the rail every few seconds.

The paramedic speaks into a radio and turns to me. "We have an order to give him Valium. It will stop the seizure."

They give him Valium but it doesn't stop the seizure. They give him more Valium, but the twitching continues. Every few seconds there is another jerk.

We get to the hospital and into the emergency room and the automatic doors swing open like they know we are coming. I recognize a nurse. She wears a pink smock and covers her mouth with her hand. There is a universal expression for fear and she has it.

A doctor appears and turns to me and says, "We'll give him more medication. It will stop the seizure." I give him Dr. Garrison's note and he tucks it in his pocket. He medicates Porter four times in all. I count. Everything is about to get worse.

The seizure doesn't stop. Two hours pass and the room is filled with doctors, one is on the phone with a specialist at the Minneapolis Children's Hospital. When he gets off, he calls me into the hall.

"We need to transport him to Children's as they are better equipped to deal with this," he says. "I am going with you."

"You're going to drive over to the other hospital?" I am both touched and scared by the customer service.

"We are going to take him by ambulance and I will ride inside with you. We need to have a doctor with him on the ride." I want to ask questions, but we don't have time. Porter's bed is wheeled out through the emergency entrance to a waiting ambulance by the door where we arrived.

The paramedics hold open the back doors as the doctor wheels Porter's stretcher towards the vehicle. We climb inside and sit on little benches across from each other. Porter twitches between us. *Jolt. Jolt. Jolt.* The doctor watches the numbers on a machine that measures Porter's oxygenation. The numbers seem big but actually are low and indicate that he is not getting what he needs from his breathing.

The doctor looks at the paramedic and says, "Saturation is sixty and I need you to pull over!" They stop the ambulance and he sticks a tube up Porter's nose and the number barely budges. We begin to drive again, faster. *Jolt.* Sirens blare. *Jolt.* The numbers on the machine go up slightly.

"I am so sorry," I say. I don't know why I say this.

"It's not for you to apologize," the doctor offers.

I touch Porter's arm. *Jolt.* The doctor does not look at me. "This must be a terrible part of the job," I say.

"This must be a terrible part of parenting," he responds. We don't say anything more.

When we arrive to Children's we are wheeled through automatic doors. More doctors meet us and the one I rode with whispers to them as they lean their heads in a circle. A half an hour after we arrive, the seizure stops.

The floors are cement. That's why all the nurses wear tennis shoes. My heels click against the ground, so I try to walk softly and drag my feet to do it. I sit next to Porter and he doesn't move. I touch his back and he doesn't move. I walk down the hall and into the lounge. I dig in my pockets, looking for some spare change, and buy a Diet Coke but don't drink it. It is morning, I think, but I can't tell for sure because I can't see outside. I get up again and walk to the parents' lounge and look through the magazines stacked in the corner. I want someone here to talk to. I want to share my dreams, but my dreams are gone. My dreams are gone because we're back in the hospital.

I continue to walk around, pacing in a tight circle. The parents' lounge has carpet so my heels don't click. There is a stain in the corner where someone has vomited. I stare at the stain and wonder about the person that left it. I wonder if their dreams are gone too. I wonder if that's why they vomited.

There is a cross above the refrigerator but it doesn't do the trick. I've always believed that there is both a visible and an invisible realm, but right now the concrete world is the only thing I can fathom. The visible is sterile and white except for where someone has vomited.

The doctors come in to tell us we must resume the seizure medication and raise the dose. They tell us what to do but not what will happen.

"You'll need to get a helmet as soon as you leave," they add. Seizures are unpredictable and he might crack his skull. I cringe at the thought of Porter in a helmet. I cringe that I cringe because the doctors are right.

I bring my articles with me to cram for a test and read the studies as I sit next to my son in the ICU. His crib has blue bumpers. They are squishy so he doesn't hurt his arms when they whap during seizures.

Today I review an experiment titled "View Through a Window May Influence Recovery from Surgery." They study the healing affect of viewing nature post-surgery. The article compares the outcomes for people with a bucolic scene and those that stare at cement buildings. The author's summary indicates that the view we have influences our emotional state and ultimate recovery.[9]

Ironically, I am the case and the study. I can see the relevance of the article in the way the hospital setting affects me. I wonder how the physical space colors my mood and the way it affects my sense of hope. I imagine my son spending formative years in cribs that have bars like jail cells. I imagine how he might feel waking up and staring through the bars. I can't stop thinking that Porter is growing up in a cage.

We spend day after day in the hospital and it is a gray, monotone landscape. I look over at my son. He is motionless. Hours later he is still asleep.

Porter receives so much Valium that he doesn't wake up for thirty-six hours. I wander down the hall to the parents' lounge again. The window faces the brick wall of the adjacent building. I don't know what time it is. The air conditioner whirs and

9 Roger S. Ulrich, "View through a window may influence recovery from surgery." *Science*, no. 224 (1984): 420–22.

the nurse is wearing a sweater. I have a coat on and it is mid-July. Without outside light it is always the same time inside.

In my neuropsychology classes I learned that the hippocampus holds our memories of location, as it integrates the information from the visual and auditory cortexes and assimilates the data in what are called "place cells." The hippocampus stamps our emotional memories and captures every scent and sight associated with them, as if to say, "This is important. Remember all these details." My memory is triggered by soap and stained carpet. *Stamp.*

It is not just smells or views that affect me. The halls are closed and white. Each one is identical. The doors slide open with a *whoosh* as I approach. Research shows that hospital settings are stressful because of the way they are designed. The layout is primed for medical efficiency and plotted so that diagnostic tools are nearby. The design is obscure for the patients, but mental health doesn't factor in efficiency. The trouble lies in a few things that trigger the stress response: the number of decision points, the threatening machines, the lack of visual cues so that the majority of time is spent lost and fumbling.

The late Irish poet John O'Donohue wrote about the way our outer environment mirrors our internal one and now it amplifies my thought: *I am lost and fumbling.*

After three days in the ICU, Porter comes home. He is dopey from drugs and loaded daily with new ones. It isn't just phenobarbital anymore—now he's taking Mysoline as well and we've gotten the pep talk that there is no end in sight. Porter may be on drugs forever. I want to know if we've hit rock bottom or if this is just a pit stop. I want to stop digging.

"Many people are on seizure medications forever and they lead very normal existences," the doctor says during our last meeting. This has come to be good news.

"You don't think he'll outgrow this?" I can't help it. I am worried about the drugs and what they will do to his developing brain.

"He might. But after the last two long seizures, I think that anoxia or dying in a protracted event is a bigger risk than taking the medications." He is in a hurry so we are done talking. I want to ask him how soon the kids outgrow the seizures and how much of a risk the drugs carry. I want to ask him why he mentioned death and then walked away. But I don't and instead we pack up Porter's belongings, grab his new prescriptions, and head back to our lives.

When we get home, Porter is in his bed with the breathing monitor again. Nonetheless I spend the night in the living room so that I can hear him if he seizes. We live in what Minnesotans call "a story-and-a-half" house. The original structure was 1,000 square feet, and the previous owner revamped the attic into a roomy space with a walk-in closet and bathroom on one end. The main floor is a square: one side with our living room and kitchen and the other end with two tiny bedrooms. We've put the kids in bunk beds on the left with Tyler on the top and Porter on the bottom. The room is packed with shelves that Brian made and filled with picture books that we read every night. They are cramped with stories since my mother signed us up for a club that sends boxes of books every month.

At 2:00 a.m., Tyler appears. She appears most nights, as she has started wandering around the house hours after going to bed. I know she's there because I feel her, breathing over my face and staring at me.

"Don't sleep on the couch!" she yells. "Sleep upstairs with Daddy!" I try to explain and she is unmoved and I finally pull her down to sleep beside me. She says immediately, "Don't close your eyes."

I pull the cover up over the two of us. She pats my back. "This is Mommy."

"This is sleeping," I say and shut my eyes again.

She isn't deterred. "Mommy's not really sleeping!"

Tyler is awake, jacked up on household tension. I give in, sit up, and turn on the light. Tyler turns to the coffee table and hands me a book. It's a new one called *Scuffy the Tugboat*. I crack it open. Reading to Tyler is a long process because she interrupts during each page to commentate on the action. Tonight is different. We get near the end, and Scuffy is stranded and it's obvious things could go several directions. Tyler snaps the book shut.

"What about the ending?" I ask.

"Time to sleep," she declares. I find myself arguing. I want to know if Scuffy is rescued or sinks, but instead we pull the blanket over us and she drifts off.

I have noticed a shift in Tyler and I worry about her every day. She is watching us closely, always hovering nearby. She is like a tiger mom to her brother. *You don't need to mother him*, I frequently tell her. *I need to watch out for him,* she'll often say back. I wonder if anyone will emerge from this story well.

I know that I add to Tyler's anxiety. I am creating experiences where she sees that things don't always follow through the way they are supposed to. I notice this the next day when we head to the library. We are out of new books at home. Not for Porter—he would have me read *Spot* seventeen times in a row, but Tyler flies through her books.

The kid section is on the left, past the sitting area with the magazines. I pick up a copy of *Dog Fancy* and read about Golden Retrievers. Tyler gets a handful of books and we stand in line by the checkout desk. Above the scanner is a sign taped to the wall and I see our name.

"Why do they have your name up there, Mommy?"

"Oh, it must be someone else." I don't really look because Porter is now under the desk.

"It says 'Sarah Bridges' and that's you." I look and see she is right. My name is up there under a note that says No more checkouts. Speak to librarian. It's exactly like gas stations that copy and post pictures of bad checks.

"I'll ask her. Don't worry, honey," I tell her. Now Tyler is twitching too, craning to read the small print below my wanted poster.

"It says, 'five books—one year late.' I think you're in trouble." I am irritated that she learned to read so early.

"Got it, thanks Tyler." I am holding Porter, who is hanging on to my hand and swinging because he won't stand up. His helmet bumps the desk as he swings back and forth.

We move to the front of the line. Tyler steps forward. She points to the note on the wall. "That's my mother, she's right here," then she points to me.

"Yes, that's me. Do we have something overdue?"

The librarian looks at the note, then at me. Porter's helmet bumps against the desk.

"Let me just look this up," she says. I hand her my library card. She makes a clucking sound. Her eyebrows go up and then the corners of her mouth turn down; 95 percent of communication is nonverbal and every bit of this message seems bad.

"We have a little problem," she says, emphasizing the last two words. Her words say little problem, but her face says big problem. She types again in the computer and then says in a stern whisper, "We can't loan you any more books."

"Do I have something overdue?" I ask again.

"You have five things that are a year overdue. Have you received the notices?"

"I probably did, I'm sorry, why don't I pay the fine now?" I let go of Porter's hand to reach in my purse and he falls on the ground and yelps.

Porter howls. The librarian clucks.

"Did you *steal* the books?" Tyler asks.

Porter screams.

"I'm afraid we are well past fines as it appears there are other missing books. I'm afraid you are on probation," the librarian says and stares at me.

Tyler clucks. Porter kicks the desk. "Oh sure, how much?" I ask.

"It will be $36 for the late fees and $54 if you don't find those five books that are still out." I pull money out of my wallet and pay her. We take our new books. I make a mental note to look for the ones we now own.

Tyler is still concerned. She leans over the counter. "How serious is it?"

"It's under control, Ty. Let's go." I get my change and grab Porter. Tyler trails a few feet behind us then stops. She runs back to the librarian.

"Will you ever take the sign down?" She is pointing at my library card up on the wall. It's clear a lot of therapy lies ahead. I grab her hand. The three of us walk through the lobby and out the glass doors.

"Why didn't you return their books, Mom?"

"I just missed the due date," I explain to her.

"You really should be on time," she says.

"The important thing is to be courteous with authority when you are in trouble." I say this to her although I can't imagine her ever running afoul of the cops. Tyler mulls this over. It strikes me that I may be teaching the wrong lesson. I imagine her being stopped by the police and saying, "Yes sir, that was my bong."

"I'd rather not get in trouble," she says.

"I'll work on it."

We get in the car and drive home. I unload Porter from his car seat and Tyler jumps out of the car. She spies our neighbor in her yard, raking, and runs over to her. As I get closer I hear her say, "My mother was banned from the library." I give a little wave to the neighbor.

That night Tyler comes to our room and flips on the overhead light. I think she must think it is morning. Or maybe her sleep cycle is off because our life is haphazard.

"Porter is having a seizure," she announces. I was up too late finishing my dissertation and I can't follow what is happening. I think Tyler is confused and so I tell her to go back to bed.

"Get up Mom and Dad!" she yells at us. I get up but it feels like my feet are on backwards. I trip and fall on my knees. When I am up, I run out of the room.

She is right. Porter is seizing. His hands are curled in and my mind flashes to an image of Karen Anne Quinlan before they pulled the plug. Brian gets there first. We lift him out of his bed and bring him to the living room to time the event.

"It's 2:03," Brian says. He unhooks his watch and holds it in front of us. We watch the hands on the clock as if we are timing a race.

"It's 2:05," he says. The neurologist wants us to call the paramedics if the seizure goes past five minutes. The hands creep around. This is the part I hate. He seizes. The hands creep. The skin around his mouth is pale blue since seizures cause anoxia. The anoxia causes brain damage if it goes on too long. It is now 2:08 and we've hit the mark. The mark is bad news and we pick up the phone.

I call 9-1-1. Then we wait. 2:12. People used to believe that you held down a person's tongue when they seized, but this is wrong. No wooden spoon, no bite board, just sitting and watching as we wait for the ambulance.

The fire truck comes first. There is no siren since it's the middle of the night, but I hear the heavy brakes and I am relieved when the firemen burst through the door. Their blue coveralls and big biceps calm me and one kneels down to give him oxygen.

"It'll be okay, Porter." They call him by name because they know him. They've been here the last two times. The men look bleary and tired and I see how bloodshot their eyes are.

It's their empathy that makes me cry. The Dalai Lama says that his religion is kindness, and if these firemen were followers they'd be zealots. Each time they come I expect one to say, "You don't seem to be getting the hang of this," when they see us. No one does. They are kind.

When things are stripped away, kindness is all that counts.

I find Tyler in her room holding her stuffed zebra. She is wearing one gray sock and underwear. I grab her hand and lead her back to the living room. She has no pants and my husband is on the couch with his head in his hands. Things are stripped away, and I don't care about my child in one sock and I don't care about the mess in the kitchen. The veneer is peeled back and I am left to cope. I am left with just the vow to make things better and get from here to there.

The seizure jolts on and the fireman talks on the phone. He says, "Got it," and they pull out a plastic syringe to give Porter a dose of Valium rectally. I look at Brian and he looks back and I turn away.

Porter jolts. There is no stretcher. The biggest fireman picks him up and cradles him against his chest and carries him outside to the ambulance. He is saying something to my son very quietly.

I ride in the ambulance next to the paramedic and he talks on the phone with the doctor, "More Valium." 2:18. Valium. 2:23. Valium. Hospital. IV of Valium. 3:17.

Then, the seizure stops.

After this episode, Porter's phenobarbital dose is doubled in an attempt to control his seizures. When this doesn't work, a new drug is then added and there still isn't a dent. We try seven different drugs and daily Valium. Nothing. Each week we check Porter's blood to see if the medication level is right. We raise the dose after each seizure. Dr. Garrison says we'll find the right recipe. There are medical solutions to most cases of epilepsy. No recipe works for us. It's as if Porter's injury lies out of bounds.

Seizure, seizure, seizure.

We are in and out of the hospital, sometimes on the same day. During one visit, the evening nurse doesn't know that we ever checked out.

My father flies out to see us. He has always been my mentor, guiding me in both writing and in work. He is also the person I turn to when things become tough.

The first morning he is at my house, we sit in the dining room and drink coffee and talk.

"What should I do, Dad?" My father is the type of person who knows something about everything. Once when I was little, I debated my friend about whether zebras were black with white stripes, or white with black stripes. Dad leaned over the newspaper and said, "Technically zebras are black with white stripes. If you shave one it will be totally black."

"Sometimes there are circumstances where there isn't a best way you can change something, Sar," he says. "Sometimes it's about how gracefully you accept what is happening." I know this is right when he says it, but it isn't something I am able to do yet. You might even say that acceptance isn't my strong suit.

I'd stopped trying to figure out how he knew these things, or how he studied Latin as his second language in high school, which is why he sprinkled in mystifying comments like, "Porter's injury is a case of 'auribus teneo lupum'"—a quote from the Roman writer Terence, and a proverb in Ancient Rome that means there is no good solution. It actually translates to "holding a wolf by the ears," or the normal person's non-Latin version, "holding a tiger by the tail." My father's wisdom typically provoked as many questions as it answered.

7

ONE YEAR

We first filed Porter's case in vaccine court six months ago and the medical records are in. But there is a glitch. Our records aren't complete.

"We need one more test," Katherine says. "They need to run a metabolic screen to be sure his seizures aren't caused by a pre-existing condition."

I know the rule-out routine; we've run blood tests, EEGs, MRIs, and genetic profiling. The process drags on. We turn in one test and then the government needs a new one. Each is negative. Basically, we do a lot of things over.

The metabolic screen seems simple enough and I go to the lab to get the materials.

I see another woman at the lab named Krissy who I met at the intensive care unit in the parents' lounge sitting under the cross. We ate Chinese takeout together and walked to the hospital pharmacy to pick up our drugs. Her son also had a brain injury when he was hit by a car while riding his bike. He awoke a day later but couldn't remember his name. She was worried that he would miss three weeks of classes. I wonder if he is back to normal.

I spot her in the lab, waiting for her child's turn, and I am unable to talk. Then we're hugging and we can't stop talking. There is a relief in speaking with someone else who has experienced this, like coming up for air after being too long underwater. I've only met her once, but it feels safe to let down my guard with her since she understands what this is like. It's the same story we always tell: We were in the hospital and it was bad, now we're out and things are good. We stand like that, half-hugging and blocking the line for the welcome desk, until we leave.

The lab tech calls us in to meet with him and hands me a plastic baggie. He is wearing a T-shirt with a slouching monkey on it and a saying that reads, "Is it Friday yet?" I'm slouching down, exhausted. I take the baggie and put it in my purse.

"Real easy," he says. "You just tape this bag over his penis and wait for him to go. Then you pour the urine in this glass vial and freeze it immediately. *Don't let it defrost!* Or we start over." His voice is stern, but his eyes are soft and I want to reassure him that I'm on top of things.

"It sounds like we're handling nuclear weapons," I joke. He doesn't get it.

"Don't worry, it's not that toxic," he says and pats my shoulder. I can tell he is worried about me. I get that a lot.

He waits for me to respond but I don't, so he repeats himself, "Real easy." It sounds real easy to me, too.

The minute we're home I start the process and strip off Porter's diaper to attach the bag. I tape it on and Porter pulls it off. He hands it to me.

I call Tyler. "Pin down his arms." Tyler holds his arms down but he wriggles free and pulls off the tape. The bag falls under the couch. The dog comes over and grabs it and I pull it out of her mouth.

"I don't think he wants to do this, Mom," Tyler says.

"He *has* to wear it. Pin him down again."

This time Tyler pulls his arms over his head and sits on them. Porter screams. I tape on the bag and close his diaper. This works for two minutes until Porter pulls off his diaper. The baggie is dangling between his legs.

"I guess he doesn't want a bag taped to his penis, Mom."

"It's taped around his penis," I tell her and she holds his arms again.

"No!" says Porter, sitting under Tyler.

"Sorry Porter, for some reason Mom wants to tape something to your privates."

I shut the diaper tighter and three hours later we have our sample. I take it into the kitchen, pack it up like the lab tech instructed, and freeze it.

Later that day, I pack the sample in a bag of ice before we head out to the doctor's office. I look outside the dining room window. It is ninety degrees and humid.

I am paranoid the ice will melt. I load the kids into the minivan to drive to the neurologist. I run a red light, somebody honks and I drive even faster since we can't do this over. I have one hand on the steering wheel and one on the sample between my legs, nestled in a bag of ice that is turning to water. We park, get out of the car, and Tyler stops with her hands on her hips.

"You're not in the white lines," she points out to me.

"I know Tyler, we need to hurry."

"You ran a red light. Are you going to get arrested?"

I get to the elevator and the bag is sloshy, I notice it has leaked and stained my crotch. A family steps on and smiles, then looks at my pants. "It's a urine sample," I say, and they stare without smiling, which strikes me as rude.

"The police are arresting my mother," Tyler says and the family steps back.

Porter flaps. I scoop him up and we run down the hall.

The nurses' station is backed up and I'm antsy, holding the bag of water up over everyone's head. "We're losing it!" I say loudly.

"We're all losing it," says the father in front of me, holding his helmeted baby. The clinic is filled with helmets and people who've lost it and Porter is grabbing coffee cups and throwing them at a girl in a wheelchair. The girl picks one up and throws it back and Porter plays catch while I butt in the line.

"Urine is everywhere," I say loudly and this does the trick. A woman in back sees the vial and slips around the counter to grab it.

We jog it down the hall to a room in the back stacked with tiny trays. We are in a windowless room with a tiny refrigerator, like the kind in dorm rooms. She slips the vial into the holder, shoves it to the back of the freezer, and hands me a towel for my pants. We'll hear back in two weeks.

We get the results. Everything is normal.

Aside from the test results, we turn in the receipts to provide proof that we've spent more than $1,000 for out-of-pocket services.

Brian and I sit at the dining table sorting through a manila folder with copies of our bills. There are the ambulance rides, hospital co-pays, medication tabs, equipment bills, and more. The folder is an inch thick. I think wistfully of the $1,000 tally, which made us qualify to file a claim after the first visit. I've come to both hate and love the sight of an ambulance. I associate it with rescue, help, and $912. That is what our last ride cost when the paramedics took Porter back to the hospital. I hate to think of money and I don't. Then I do when our bank account is overdrawn.

Brian holds up the pile of bills at me, "Do you think we qualify?"

Finally we have the medical records and the out-of-pocket payments. Our co-pays and out-of-network visits pile up and we keep the stack of bills on the counter near the phone. The breathing monitor has a monthly rental charge and every lab visit runs up a tab. There is no money since I only have the scholarship I'm given for graduate school. We've run through our cash and hold off on fixing our refrigerator. Water seeps out from the bottom of the door and one of us slips in it every day. We wait to fix it because we believe that the end is near, that help is so close. Our file is complete and we wait for the special court to render its verdict. For now, I have dish towels blocking the gap of the door where the water seeps out. *I can do this for ninety days*, I think.

But after three months, the refrigerator still leaks.

We go another month after that. Then the government asks for a 120-day extension to review all the testing. I wonder what they were doing during the previous four months. We wait another six weeks. Katherine says the government moves slowly. This is a race and we are all tortoises.

After yet another month Katherine calls with some news. "The government has asked for an extension as they feel you need an extended EEG."

"A what?"

"You'll need to go to Gillette's Specialty Hospital and check Porter in for three days. They'll wire his scalp and he'll have a continuous EEG. The hope is that they'll capture seizure activity. The government is arguing that he has a pre-existing condition causing the seizures."

"I thought we answered that with all the tests we've done."

"One more," she says. "Then we'll be done."

The continuous EEG monitors electrical activity over a period of time. The idea is that the mound of data generated will pinpoint inconclusive seizure activity and highlight the origin. It is touted as one part of the best lineup aimed at identifying brain injury.

A week later we have confirmation from the hospital. Porter will be checked in and wear an electrode cap for three days to see if we can find ground zero for his seizures. The outcome sounds promising. The seventy-two-hour part sounds iffy.

When I call about our visit that afternoon I go over everything with a nurse. We will check into the hospital the next morning and be asked to review preparation.

"Just keep him up the night before," the nurse says.

"He goes to bed at half past eight. How do you recommend doing that? Should I give him coffee?" This is a joke, but she doesn't get it.

"You should *never* give a toddler coffee. How long have you been doing that?" I can picture her shaking her head. I have the feeling she thinks we could skip the EEG because she's discovered the cause of his seizures.

"We don't give him coffee, that was just a joke," I respond, but she doesn't laugh. Papers shuffle.

"All righty then." This is Minnesotan speak for "up yours."

I hang up the phone and plan for the evening. I make a pot of coffee. It's all for me.

I am awake when Tyler calls me to her room.

"My stomach hurts," she says. I am certain it is psychosomatic because of the stress. Then I worry that I am becoming my mother, always analyzing things.

I put her to bed and tell her sleep will help. I get a bowl from the kitchen and place it on the floor beside her bed. Five minutes later she calls me back to her room. She is sitting up and her stuffed horse and teddy bear are in the bowl. I pull her out of the bed and start to prepare her a bath. Behind me I hear Porter's noisy breathing as he sleeps curled up on the side of the bed. I brace myself for a long night.

Gillette Children's Hospital sits in downtown St. Paul and caters to young patients with disabilities. A specialty here is epilepsy and it is the best place in the area to have a protracted EEG.

The ride to the hospital is tortuous as Porter nods off in his car seat and Tyler shrieks at the top of her lungs, "*No sleeping*

Porter!" Then I scream at Tyler to stop screaming at Porter. She screams, I scream, he sleeps.

We arrive early and are sent up a bank of elevators to a special wing where these tests are done. Inside I see a common space populated by toddlers and older children playing with toys. It's a normal scene, save the wires: Each child is connected to a tangle of cords that trail behind them everywhere they go.

A nurse checks us in and directs us to a room that Porter will share with another boy. He sits in his bed rocking, clutching a fabric softener bottle. His mother looks up and waves and I wave back. The boy rocks.

Porter flaps and bangs on his helmet. The other boy yells.

"I'm sorry," she says. "He's very distressed by noise."

Porter bangs. Roommate screams. I nod.

The first step is the fitting. This sounds fun, like trying on a wedding dress, but it's not fun and feels more like getting a tooth pulled. I have a flashback to our last visit to Great Clips when we had to leave halfway through Porter's haircut because he kept trying to grab the scissors.

The first step is to attach the cap. We follow a technician into a special room where she approaches Porter with a red felt pen.

"Hey buddy, we're going to draw little Xs on your head." Porter ignores her and lies under the exam table. I'm fairly certain he's licking the floor. "I just need you up here on the table for a few minutes. It won't hurt, I promise."

I manage to hold Porter as she begins the process. She puts a tape measure around his skull like a headband and marks something down in her notes. Then she marks designated spots. For the first few minutes Porter laughs because he thinks it's funny. Or because he remembers something funny. Or maybe he's having a psychotic episode. After fifteen minutes, the novelty wears off and I restrain Porter using the basket-hold technique of pinning his arms to his sides. As the technician marks, I squeeze, and he screams.

Attaching the electrode cap isn't any easier. It takes two of us to hold him down as we wrestle it, but the technician is unfazed and gives it a little yank to force it into place. There's no messing around. I like this woman.

"These things are indestructible. This is the fidget-proof version," she says.

"Is there something to the right of the fidget one? Maybe a combat version?"

"It'll hold with this." She hooks a strap around his chin to keep it in place. Porter screams. He looks like an angry swimmer.

I lift him down and he bolts out of the room, but is stopped by the tether attached to the cap. It's exactly like having him on a leash, only this one is attached to the top of his head and gives a snap when he runs too far. He tries to yank it off and can't and lies on the floor crying.

I look at my watch. Only seventy-one and a half hours to go.

I have the first shift and Brian has the second. Someone needs to be at the hospital with Porter. We can't explain to him why he's there, or why he has to wear a tight-fitting hat that he hates, or why his roommate wails all night and I act like nothing is weird.

He never gets used to the cap. He runs, it snaps, and he grabs his scalp. This happens for six hours: run, snap, grab.

I look at the other mothers and I notice that they act like nothing is odd. I think about these strangers who don't have the range of reactions they ought to have. They look like refrigerator mothers.

When Brian arrives, I meet him at the door. I've been up since 2:00 a.m. and have drunk four cups of black coffee. I am not the best version of myself.

"How did it go?" he asks. He looks rested and normal.

"Well, he hates the cap, can't pull it off, and is homicidal. Otherwise, he's great."

"Okay. I brought in *Winnie the Pooh*. The brochure said they have video machines."

"Good luck," I say, pointing to the fabric softener bottle boy. "His roommate doesn't like noises and shrieks when he hears them. Apparently he doesn't sleep at night."

Porter looks at Brian and pulls on his sleeve.

"Okay," is all Brian says.

After his seventy-two-hour EEG, the results come in. "Porter has disorganized electrical activity in his brain," the neurologist tells us as we sit on Porter's bed. The doctor wears a button-down shirt and Dockers and has a clamp-on teddy bear affixed to his tie. He looks well rested.

"I was fairly certain this was true before we had our visit," I say. I am not trying to be rude; I'm trying to be funny. But it comes out curt since I am also insane at this point. The doctor pretends he doesn't notice.

"We captured several events as he slept and can see that they emanate from the left side of his brain. We don't see anything else that sheds much light on the etiology of his seizures." The neurologist says he'll talk with our neurologist and share the news that we have no news. We also send the results to the government. No news should be good news, but in our case no news means more tests.

We've been back to the ICU twelve times so far and our bills rack up. We are lucky to have insurance, but insurance only pays for a portion of costs. Each hospital stay results in a flurry of charges: the ambulance, doctors, medications, supplies, anesthesiology, specialists, and EMTs. Our visits occur so close together that our balances at the hospitals are often confused because insurance response is delayed—bills are out of date by the time we try to pay them. Or maybe it's the fact that we don't have money to pay them.

The compensation for vaccine injuries occurs on promissory notes and we log our medical bills in a notebook by the phone. The attorney's fees are dealt with similarly: Lawyers that work on the claims are paid at the end if the case is won. This seemed feasible in the 240-day scenario the program promised, but the six-month plan never happens. Our lawyer files claims and writes briefs all in the belief that the bills will be paid when the settlement is received. In the meantime, Katherine fronts the costs for her hours, the filing fees, the records, and our experts. Another year passes. The bills pile up.

"I hate to tell you this," Katherine says when I answer the phone the following week, "but the government has pushed back the hearing saying that we haven't examined Porter for parasitic infections. I forgot to ask before, but do you have pets?"

"No pets."

"They are saying that he may have toxoplasmosis, which in turn can cause encephalitis and seizures," she tells me.

"How do you get it?"

"Usually from a cat, HIV, or after an organ transplant."

"No, no, and no. Does that settle it?"

"We need to have him get some blood work done. Luckily there is a test for antibodies."

"That's it? Just one more test?" I ask, trying to feel hopeful.

"That's what they are saying."

"Got it." I'm feeling frustrated, yet again.

"You're doing great!" Katherine offers me some encouragement before hanging up.

We test Porter for toxoplasmosis. He is negative for antibodies. That's two in the win column: no toxoplasmosis and he still has all of his organs.

Months pass. Despite his daily seizures, Porter took his first step soon after his first birthday. Porter's abilities are funny this way—some things are in perfect order while other things are blown to bits. A year after the step, he mumbles his first word. I am in shock.

I tap Tyler's shoulder and ask her, "Did you hear that? He just said a word."

"Yeah! It sounded like *mutton*," she responds.

"It wasn't *mutton*, it was *momma*. Porter, say it again."

He ignores me, turning back to refill his letter puzzle. For the next twenty minutes I try to coax him to talk. Nothing.

"I know I heard it," I say to Tyler. Even I can see how weird it is that I am so bent on convincing a four-year-old.

"Yeah, he said it," she agrees finally. "But Mom, why does he call you *mutton*?"

I keep track of these milestones in a spiral notebook, physical evidence that Porter is doing well. One afternoon several months later, I sit on the floor of the basement playroom as Tyler and Porter build LEGO towers. I am ready to take notes.

"Tyler, help me think of all the words that Porter knows," I ask her. I'd just read the chapter in *What to Expect in the Toddler Years*, and knew he should have a few dozen by now. Tyler leans back and thinks for a minute.

"Like *honey*?" she asks.

"Yeah."

"And Christopher?" She is thinking hard.

"Good—keep going," I tell her.

"'Look Mom, a kite!' That's a long one that he knows."

We continue on this way for twenty minutes as I compile a numbered list. When we finish, I count the words and smile to myself when we get to one hundred. He is above average. Then it hits me: aside from some favorite foods in the list, all of the words that Porter speaks are phrases from his *Winnie the Pooh* videos.

The things he says echo what he hears. This is called echolalia. I find it endearing in small doses, but often less lovable when he repeats himself for an hour.

Running one morning with Porter in the baby jogger, he starts saying, "Stupid head, stupid head, stupid head," in a monotone voice. I try to ignore it, jogging faster, hoping the runner's high will kick in. But twenty minutes later he is still at it. "Stupid head," I hear from below me.

Finally I've had enough. I stop the jogger, get down on one knee, and lean in close to him. "Stop saying that, Porter, it isn't nice." There is a pause as I stand back up and start running again.

A minute later I hear below me, "Dummy head."

I still count the words. After all, the toddler book says repeating things is how babies learn.

Although I know Porter is different than most kids his age, his disability is broadcast to the world by his helmet, it announces *seizures* everywhere we go. Each day the seizures occur in some variation: grand mal or petite mal. They happen in public and they happen at home.

Porter's helmet also broadcasts something else: vulnerability that is featured and unapologetic. His vulnerability exemplifies the Latin root *vulnera,* which means "to wound." I know intellectually that everyone has emotional soft spots. Most of us just hide them better. Instead, Porter's wound is worn on the outside like a seahorse's skeleton. The defenselessness he has affects people in a way that I only begin to comprehend when he is older. I am slowly starting to understand that God didn't cause this to happen to Porter. God is present in the way we respond to things we can't fix.

8

18 MONTHS

Our life occurs in medical chapters. It is unpredictable because seizures are unpredictable. The shot caused a problem because vaccines have side effects; when I signed the release, I understood this. I embrace the notion I learned at my liberal arts college of *public good,* or a shared benefit that pertains to all of us. However, public good can have private shortfalls, and sometimes what edifies the group decimates the individual. I embrace the good that vaccines have provided to millions of people. I understand that when millions of people take a drug, there will be some that respond unfavorably. But it only seems fair to take care of those children.

I understood the risk when I vaccinated my son, but I can't comprehend the lack of acknowledgment of our family's casualty. I am not looking for the government to undo what has happened; I am merely looking for someone to acknowledge it. There is an extensive body of research about the simple effect that a doctor's apology has on the outcome of medical errors.[10]

10 Jennifer K. Robbennolt, "Apologies and Medical Error." *Clinical Orthopaedics and Related Research* 467, no. 2 (2009): 376–82.

Much of the data comes later and says that acknowledgment is critical in the process of coming to terms with the mistake.

No one apologizes about Porter and no one says there was harm done. It is only years later that I read the work of Dr. Robbennolt in which she states, "Apologies—statements that acknowledge an error and its consequences, take responsibility, and communicate regret for having caused harm—can decrease blame, decrease anger, increase trust, and improve relationships. Importantly, apologies also have the potential to decrease the risk of a medical malpractice lawsuit and can help settle claims by patients."[11] No one meant us harm, but they did do harm. In the absence of apology, the injury leads to insult. It leads to a void filled with confusion and anger and ambiguity. It is silent and unpredictable and lonely.

I keep expecting validation when I see our pediatrician. We see her every month and we pretend we have no history. We never talk about the first night he was hospitalized, or what the ER doctor said, or that she came in to see us at 3:00 a.m. She doesn't know what to say or how to say it, so instead she pretends that nothing happened.

I know about the research on forgiveness. I took the Transgression Narrative Test of Forgivingness (TNTF) that John Berry and Everett Worthington created in the course of a psychology class. It is a survey that describes various scenarios and asks you to rate the likelihood that you'd forgive the offender in each. I think of it now and remember what it showed. Your totaled scores reveal your dispositional forgiveness, something that is correlated with a personality trait called agreeableness. My score says my default setting is acceptance. My default is to move past any grudge about what happened.[12]

11 Ibid.

12 Jack W. Berry et al., "Dispositional Forgivingness: Development and Construct Validity of the Transgression Narrative Test of Forgivingness (TNTF)." *Personality and Social Psychology Bulletin* 27, no. 10 (2001): 1277–290.

It is not different now. I accept that medications carry risk and that the small percent in the *serious side effect* category are things called injured humans. I accept, almost from the start, that the event happened. What I can't accept is that there is no one on the other side of our injury claim reaching a hand across to apologize. There is no one from the government reaching out to us and acknowledging that a casualty occurred.

Sister Helen Prejean says anger is a moral response, and all of us feel it when we are hurt. She is a nun who works with death row convicts, and the author of *Dead Man Walking*.

I know from brain studies that we are wired to lash out when somebody hurts us. From a neuropsychological perspective, the revenge-seeking brain looks like that of someone that is starving and poised to eat. When we visualize our revenge, the rewards center of the brain lights up in a loop, almost like a string of Christmas lights. I understand this urge to strike back.

We go to the doctor every week. I sit in the waiting area on the floor next to the LEGO table. There are kid-sized chairs and ratty books. Mothers and babies are next to me and I look at them, wondering if any of them have ever thought their children might stop breathing before the ambulance arrives. The nurse that checks me in looks at Porter's chart and asks how long he's had seizures. Maybe she's new, or maybe the process is new, or maybe there isn't a process. I smile and give my spiel as Porter pulls the paper sheet off the examining table.

"Looks like the seizures started at four months," she says, reading from the chart.

"On the day he got eight vaccines," I add.

"Oh, vaccines don't have side effects," she informs me.

"Then why do we sign the release saying vaccines have side effects?" I ask her.

She looks up and a smile creeps onto the corners of her mouth.

"For liability reasons," she replies.

"But you said there are no side effects," I point out.

"There aren't."

That's it, I give up. She doesn't know I've read about the pertussis vaccine. She doesn't know I love research and study the subject daily in the medical library at the University of Minnesota.

The nurse weighs Porter and takes his vitals. I don't push the topic any further with her. I don't want to sound paranoid.

There are so many things I could say. What I've learned in my coursework crosses my mind. Aside from the neuropsychological testing I do in the medical school, I also work with animals in the lab. In this context I've encountered something called EAS, or "experimental autoimmune encephalomyelitis." It is a way of inducing brain inflammation, usually in rodents, to explore various human diseases. The animals are rendered disabled when they are injected with poison. Pertussis toxin is a favorite as it induces brain injury in rats and mice during experimentation. Pertussis toxin was injected into my son when he was four months old. It was only nine months after his shot that the vaccination formula was changed due to safety concerns. I considered showing the nurse a printout of the information I found on the CDC website the night before but decided to walk away. The CDC's information on pertussis read:

> Whole-cell DTP vaccines are commonly associated with several local adverse events (e.g., erythema, swelling, and pain at the injection site), fever, and other mild systemic events (e.g., drowsiness, fretfulness, and anorexia) (5,6). More severe systemic events (e.g., convulsions {with or without fever} and hypotonic hyporesponsive episodes) occur less frequently (ratio of one case to 1,750 doses administered) among children who receive whole-cell DTP vaccine (5). Acute encephalopathy occurs even more rarely (ratio of 0–10.5 cases to one million doses administered). Concerns

about safety prompted the development of more purified (acellular) pertussis vaccines that are associated with a lower frequency of adverse events and are effective in preventing pertussis disease.[13]

I find the conflicting messages about the vaccine's safety stemming from the CDC and the American Academy of Pediatrics (AAP) intriguing. If anyone were to punch in the search words: *pertussis vaccine, safety,* and *adverse reactions*, over a hundred studies would appear. I think about what I read about Japan and Western Europe banning the older pertussis vaccine due to safety concerns and that it took the Food and Drug Administration (FDA) fifteen years to mandate the same for babies here.

When I was eight years old, my neighbor Paul was hit by a car. He was supposed to stay after school and at the last moment he opted to head home. He shouldn't have been on the driveway that day. He shouldn't have been killed by the car.

I came upon the scene as I walked home from school. He was lying in the street and a girl stood beside him crying hysterically. My other neighbor, a man who lived next door, knelt next to Paul, crying, and whispered something in his ear. Paul's head was bleeding and the asphalt below him was dark red. The man took his shirt off and pressed it against Paul's head. I knew he would die. Someone screamed in the background and I heard a siren approach. We kids were told a hundred times not to ride our bikes down the steep driveways into the street. In the flash of a minute, the time it takes to breathe one breath, Paul was gone.

It is less Paul's death I think of now than the reaction of his mother at the funeral. She stood next to the coffin and touched

---

13 CDC. Pertussis Vaccination: Use of Acellular Pertussis Vaccines Among Infants and Young Children Recommendations of the Advisory Committee on Immunization Practices (ACIP). MMWR March 28, 1997.

the stuffed tiger that lay under his arm. To everyone that passed she said, "He wasn't supposed to be there that day. He was supposed to be gone. If the day was just different he'd still be alive."

I think of this now as I read the documents about the timing of Porter's vaccine. It wasn't supposed to be there that day. If the day was just different, just ten months later, this never would have happened.

But it did. There is a trail of blood, but it leads back to no one.

After another month passes, Katherine contacts our special master. The government exceeded the deadline and we request a response to the filing we've made. No response occurs and we wait another month. The outcome is murky and the seizures continue. The government has another delay as they review his testing. We finally get their official response: The results of the tests we've done are too old so we must start all over. Between the official governmental response and life at home I am almost emotionally swamped.

There's a parents' seizure support group at a facility called the Courage Center and I show up, because when your child is brain damaged everyone tells you to get counseling. The facility provides therapy and living accommodations for people with disabilities. I walk from the parking lot to a small path that hugs a tiny creek. Two long-haired men in wheelchairs sit by the back door, smoking cigarettes. They meet my eyes as I walk past though neither greets me.

Inside the building the place has an industrial feel. I peek inside rooms until I find the right one. There is a picture of a man in a wheelchair shooting baskets on the wall. He is smiling from ear to ear. We sit in a circle on folding chairs and I recognize a person two seats over. Her hair is pulled back in a ponytail and her sweatshirt says, "The Black Dog Saloon." I think I know that place. I wonder if I've met her on Martha's Vineyard. I introduce myself and then realize she was in a graduate class with me a year before.

"How are you?" I ask as we sit in a circle for parents with damaged kids.

"Great!" she says, which is code for terrible. She looks terrible. I tell her she looks great. Her son has seizures and her doctor says she is depressed. My son has seizures and I am not depressed. I am high energy, which is another word for agitated. I try to connect with her, but she is staring at her purse.

The group is like a Quaker's meeting, but quieter. At first, the room is silent. It is like driving without directions. It is a parents' group but all the participants are mothers. The woman across from me is fidgeting.

Julie's hair is bobbed and curly and she wears a beeper on her belt. She breaks the ice. "I hate silence!" she says and it comes out like a cheer. I can picture the pom-poms she had in high school. "I'm a doer. I solve problems. I run the fitness program at our elementary school."

I have no idea where she is going with this and am pretty sure she wandered into the wrong group. I wonder if I should tell her. "It's my mission to make all the fat kids skinny!" she continues. The group is silent.

She looks down. "I can't explain how it feels to watch daily seizures," she says, but she tries to elaborate and the description goes on for half an hour. Her son has epilepsy. She tried to fix it and it isn't fixed. He's had seizures for over a year. "On every major holiday!" she adds. Her voice lights up at the end of each sentence, as if every statement is a question. My classmate fumbles in her purse and takes a pill. I tap my foot and stare at the happy man in the wheelchair.

The woman is still talking. Now she looks happy. Did we know that acupuncture stops seizures? "I didn't buy it when they stuck a needle in his ear. Of course, I couldn't understand her China-babble so maybe they were treating something else!" This is a joke and the woman laughs and slaps her knee. The other women near her give fake smiles on cue, like this is part of the plan. "A needle in the ear is all you need to do!"

The meeting wraps up late. I hug my classmate and she is stiff and awkward like a teenage boy. We promise to call each other. We never call.

Despite the strangeness of the meeting, I am calmed by being near people who understand so I don't need to explain my experience. It reminds me of what I've read about the tradition in Europe of passing time on train journeys by telling strangers your life story. The people in the support group are strangers, but they know my story. I want to go back. I want to stay longer.

9

TWO AND A HALF YEARS

We realize something is wrong and we want to fix it.

But it isn't that simple. The "normal" intellectual and emotional milestones for toddlers are broad enough that I can work the numbers to have Porter in the normal range. To get this validated, I see the neurologist the next week and tell him about Porter's one hundred words.

"That's great!" he says back so enthusiastically I don't have the heart to tell him what the words are.

"He still doesn't seem to understand much of what I'm saying," I continue. "I thought the comprehension part came first."

"Boys are often late. My friend's son didn't say a word until he was almost three, then two months later he knew all the presidents." I watch Porter with a puzzle and try to picture him pointing out a snapshot of Reagan and I can't do it. Instead, I pick up the tongue depressors that Porter threw at the doctor. I am wondering if the neurologist is connecting the dots that I am.

I don't say it then, but I know something deeper is wrong with Porter. I ask Dr. Garrison about autism, but he says it is too early to diagnose. Porter isn't the same as the other kids.

I know something is wrong with his speech. When Porter had his EEG, they found that his seizures emanated from the region known as *Wernicke's Area*. Damage to this part leaves gaps in receptive language, or the way we understand what others are saying. While people can still fluidly connect words, they often are out of tune and lack meaning. Knowing dozens of words doesn't count for much when they pop out at the wrong moments. Porter has damage on his left side. He doesn't use language correctly. The math is easy.

We wrap up the neurology visit with a blood-level test, and Porter and I take the elevator to the parking lot. I carry him to the car and buckle him in quickly.

"Tigger's stuck in a tree," he says. I nod. It could be worse than Winnie the Pooh.

The next day in Walgreens the cashier says, "Things happen for a reason," as I pay for another phenobarbital prescription. She wears a blue and green smock like a candy striper and a button with a boy and a baseball on it. She knows about Porter's seizures—she's kept up to date on the latest hospitalization as I see her each month. I've heard this comment and others like it before: that Porter is special, that I am special, that God plucked us out of line for being strong. Each time I nod and sometimes say thanks, because I know it is meant to help, or maybe just to make them feel a little better. It is always from well-meaning people, always from people without severely sick children. When I think of Porter unconscious or blue, pocked with needle marks and crying, I am hard-pressed to imagine these specific details are part of God's plan.

Yet, the comments do change my thinking and crystallize what I actually believe. Meaning has to come from Porter's struggle. It is my job to find that meaning and to make my reason, and in the process, to find the spirituality laced in the experience. In low points—waiting for the paramedics, holding Porter on his side as he convulses and throws up—I hang on to this idea.

The months stack on top of each other and we are willing to try anything that will help Porter's seizures. If we can't force him to hit the developmental signposts we can try to find a better medical intervention. Brian and I play good cop/bad cop with the doctors. I am enthusiastic about anything we can try while Brian is cynical it will help. Of course, Brian is right—none of the drugs have proved to be more than a speed bump for Porter's daily seizures. Yet it makes me mad that Brian isn't trying harder to be optimistic about things.

One day after another neurology appointment I say, "The doctor thinks that if we add a daily Valium it may have a good effect with the Mysoline."

"Have you noticed that his answer to everything is to raise the drugs?" Brian responds. He is right—that is what we usually do. And each time it works for a while. Porter will go a few days or even a week without a seizure and we are hopeful. Until the next seizure.

It isn't that I don't understand Brian's attitude, but rather that it scares me. It has to be bad luck to question Porter's doctors, as they are the only people who can help us. So I insist superstitiously that we only focus on the positive. It irritates me when Brian breaks the rule.

Each time we try and it fails, I see the damage reflected in Brian's face. During the next seizure a few nights later, I find Brian crying in Porter's room. I stand behind him and put my arms around his waist and we don't move. We don't talk; we can't find any words. We don't talk and a space grows between us. With each seizure, it yawns wider.

We have filed our claim and waited more than 240 days. Then the government extends the deadline and by then we have waited an entire year. We complete the metabolic screen, EEG, blood work, and genetic testing and are back at the starting line. I realize that the rule-out clause was the glitch in our case: the need to demonstrate that other things can't explain Porter's injury. The government wants proof, but only proof of what didn't happen—the kind of proof that is hard to prove.

The government says they can't meet the deadline because the data is too old. The data is too old because they've moved the deadline. I think of what Joseph Heller described as a Catch-22 when he wrote about the airman who would be crazy to fly more missions, but too sane to get out of them if he asked.

We are in a Catch-22 that Doc Daneeka would appreciate. There is no use fighting since there is no one to fight. There isn't even a specific person to get mad at.

One year into our case, the HHS lawyer changes and we are delayed again as the new person gets up to speed with our case. We begin with a second metabolic screen and twelve days later I sit across from the specialist, ready for the test results.

He begins, "I may have bad news. I've sent the urine to the University of Minnesota for analysis and one of the tests came back in the suspicious range. It's his lysine, and his level is four times above normal. That isn't just a borderline elevation—it likely means a problem. In fact, it may mean that he has lysine anemia."

I clench my teeth and smile at him. I'd like him to notice how considerate I am; surely a sign that Porter's family is the kind of people he'd like to work with. There is a lot of literature on the medical prognosis of *good* and *bad* patients. The health care professionals always prefer the good ones. It is even more complicated than that. Patients showing confidence and skill with their problems are considered *activated* and are seen as winners in managing their illness. I'm an activated winner. I hope he notices.

I take a breath. I am not quiet because I am unsure, but instead because these conversations are inherently awkward. I wonder if they ever do role-plays in medical school to teach the students how to chat with people after their kids go haywire.

"What's lysine anemia?" I ask.

"A rare metabolic disorder that causes neurological problems and, unfortunately, is terminal and incurable. We'll need to run the tests again. I will know for sure in two weeks."

I go home that night, dragging, wondering how we've gone from managing a seizure disorder to a life-threatening condition.

But two weeks later, it is all a fluke.

The doctor's voice is light as we speak on the phone one morning. "Good news! We've rerun the test and it looks fine—just a false elevation. So everything is fine. I mean, he doesn't have lysine anemia." This is win number three, but it doesn't do much for me; I've lost the ability to differentiate good and bad news since each one often disguises itself as the other.

I agree to keep track of Porter's seizures in a notebook so that we can identify whether any patterns emerge. Then we end the call and I hang up the phone.

I report this to Katherine during one of our weekly calls. "It will help the case if you gather affidavits from the people that treat Porter." I start a to-do list with one task: Get a letter from all of Porter's people. Below the heading, I add the people who have worked with Porter over the last year and who would be most helpful: our pediatric neurologist, the ER doctor, the neuropsychologist, the behavioral psychologist, the occupational therapist, the Gillette doctor, speech therapist, school evaluator, and day care teacher.

Gathering documentation is easier said than done. It is slow, despite everyone's willingness. I call each doctor's office and go through the drill, and each time it unfolds in practically the same way. I try our pediatric neurologist first. I get the call center.

"I was hoping to have Dr. Garrison write a note in support of my son's vaccine case," I tell the person on the other end.

"Dr. Garrison doesn't give vaccines, he's a neurologist," she informs me.

"Right. We see him every few weeks. He treats the seizures my son has from his vaccine injury," I explain.

"Vaccines are safe. The press out there is misinformation. I would call your pediatrician to get him immunized," she responds.

"Thanks, but too late. He is immunized. He has an injury and Dr. Garrison treats it. He said he would write a letter for our case."

"Hmm, Dr. Garrison doesn't do legal cases. He can probably refer you to someone who does that expert stuff. Have you tried calling the University of Minnesota?"

"I really appreciate your help—we don't need an expert witness per se. I'm just following up to get a letter that Dr. Garrison already said he'd be willing to write."

"I see," she says. *Tap, tap, tap.* "I'll send him a note: vaccine problems." This seems as good a description as any and I let it go. I wonder what she is typing and if there is a rider attached to files for hysterical mothers.

"Just sent it off," she tells me and we are done.

Tap, tap, tap, tap, tap.

C-R-A-Z-Y.

A month later the affidavits are in, but the government wants their own person. Katherine says they tend to seek a second opinion.

"I think you mean more like an eighth opinion?" I tell her.

"They often have their own expert give a perspective."

"They are going to fly someone to Minnesota to evaluate Porter?"

"It's more likely they will review the records and give another take."

It's hard to picture what take someone will have that the other seven people missed, but I don't say this. My first step in acceptance is to stop fighting with my allies. It's hard not to fight.

Three months later, the issue boils down to this: Porter's injury is a classic table event, and all the clinicians treating him write a letter to this effect. However, you need to pay close attention to the language and follow the cheat sheet in the government instructions, titled, "Questions and aids to Interpretation." *CliffsNotes* for discussing the vaccine injuries. It's a circular journey. We can't use a diagnosis of encephalopathy to establish a table injury of encephalopathy. Instead, we need the symptoms that lead to the diagnosis of encephalopathy. The HHS expert is concerned that the symptoms have been misinterpreted. It strikes me as odd that this mystery clinician has never spent fifteen minutes with my son, but his medical opinion carries equal weight. The government doctor wants to revisit our testing. He thinks we have missed something.

The months tick by. Any illness is tricky, and Porter catches colds constantly. The key is to keep his fever down since body temperature has an inverse correlation to the seizure threshold.

But there's an even trickier part: determining whether the fever caused seizing or the seizure caused the fever. The night we get the latest metabolic screening, we awake at 2:00 a.m. to Porter screaming. He is hot and twitching. The lights are on and the family is tense.

"Get the Advil and the thermometer!" I say, ordering Brian who is holding Tyler a few feet away. I sound aggressive and Brian runs to the bathroom without saying anything. Tyler gets up and puts a coat on over her pajamas. She waits by the door without a word.

We ride to the ER, find he has a 103-degree fever, and wait in the exam room for the results of his blood work. The seizure stops and we want to go home. At breakfast time, we leave with the advice to cycle Tylenol™ and ibuprofen over the next two days. We're told to wake up every three hours to do this and to check his temperature. That night, we stay up until midnight and set the alarm for 3:00 a.m. We oversleep by half an hour and awaken to another seizure. We head back to the clinic and test again for infection. The results are inconclusive and we start antibiotics that day. Our life is inconclusive and we wait for the response from the vaccine court.

The lack of sleep spills into every area. Reserves are low. In my neuroscience seminar the next day we talk about the perils of being sleep deprived.

"Here are my favorites," my professor says. He is a cut-to-the-chase New Yorker and he looks right at me when he tells us. "People who are chronically sleep deprived get dumb, forgetful, and fat." I make a mental run through the list of symptoms. It is the only test on which I score a 100 percent right now.

I take the kids to the park when Porter's fever is down and watch Tyler pick dandelions as Porter pours sand from cup to cup. Two women sit on the bench beside me talking in hushed voices and I strain to eavesdrop. They are discussing their husbands.

A few feet away, a child falls off the jungle gym. Other mothers leap to help and I am pleased I don't have to be the one handling it. I observe my response to the accident. It appears that I am losing my empathy and assume it is a sign of a new psychiatric diagnosis. I add the thought to my mental to-do list: one, research ways to handle sleep deprivation; two, investigate whether I have developed a personality disorder.

At the neurologist's office, he suggests we try a medication called Depakote. "It's a great drug," he says, "though it is not recommended for kids under two years old."

"Why not?" I ask, although I am unclear if I want an answer.

"Depakote can lead to liver failure and death and is off-label for kids under two. There is a definite risk in taking it so young, though my read of the research says that most of the deaths are associated with kids with more severe problems."

I look at Porter sitting in the corner hitting his helmet on the floor. I am relieved to hear there are other kids worse off. Then I catch myself. Another sign of my emerging personality disorder: lack of empathy for other sufferers.

"It's up to you and Brian if we try it, but if it were my child I would. We'll check his liver function every week, so we should catch any problem early."

I ponder this and discuss the choice with Brian. Leave things the way they are and a seizure may kill him. Stop the seizures with a new drug and the drug may kill him. We start the drug.

10

3 YEARS

Porter is three years old. He has daily seizures and goes to the hospital every few weeks. We adapt to these stints and I keep a bag packed in the hall closet like the one I had for the maternity ward. It has a toothbrush, sweatpants, and books for the hours waiting. I keep my notebook in there as well to track our progress or our lack of progress.

Our court case limps forward. We've passed each deadline and no response is forthcoming. Katherine calls to fill us in on the latest details.

"I checked in with their lawyers this morning and they said the delay is due to a missing metabolic screen."

"We did that last fall! It was normal."

"We did, and we sent it. Apparently, they've lost it and put the case on hold because the file was incomplete. I've faxed it back over and that should be the last piece." She handles this all so well.

"How can they lose it? That was the second one we ran since the first one expired."

"This happens a lot. I will stay on top of them." She is doing her best to reassure and placate me.

"So nobody calls you if something is missing?"

"I'm afraid not. They just stop the case."

"I thought this was rapid justice, in six months and all that. It's been almost two years." My patience has been wearing thin for so long now.

"I know it's frustrating, but hang in there. You have a classic case; this is just a matter of getting the information in front of the judge. In this court system he is called a special master and we are setting a date for a hearing."

I appreciate Katherine's encouragement, though it's losing its punch. The special master has taken on a mythical quality and I'm beginning to wonder if the person exists. I'm trapped in Alice's Wonderland and forced to believe as many as six impossible things before breakfast.

We set a date for the hearing. We need to travel to Washington, DC, to present our case. I want the government's doctor to join us for the journey, to have a few hours to evaluate Porter in a natural setting. I wonder if we should film the plane trip with Porter and present that as evidence. I want to sit in the court face to face with the lawyer that rejects Porter's tests and the testimonies of his physicians. But by this point there have been three new government attorneys assigned to the case. Each one steps into the role at HHS and halts our progress by asking for new evidence, and then they leave and someone new comes along with more requests. The months stretch into years. Wait and then more waiting. Our hearing approaches. Then moves. Then approaches.

Finally, help arrives. The county has a program for the *severe cases* of disability and if you qualify, they will fund part-time helpers. The Medical Assistance-TEFRA (MA-TEFRA) program is a state-funded program for kids who qualify for around-the-clock institutional care. Its aim is to keep children out of facilities by paying for supportive medical care at home.

MA-TEFRA is the Holy Grail. I know this from my support group at Courage Center. The punch line goes like this: "Everyone wants it, but no one gets it." There are either too many disabled kids or not enough money. Or disabled kids cost too much money. Whatever the case, I don't get my hopes up.

When I call the agency I'm told, "You can apply, but it will be years before you are considered." The Tibetan Buddhist saying comes to mind: *Everything preceding this event was aimed to ready you for this moment*. I'm poised.

"We still want to apply," I tell her. "We are in the swing of waiting."

A few weeks later, the Minnesota Department of Health sends a nurse to visit. She is sturdy and no-frills, a perfect icon for our state.

"I will assess Porter through a blend of observation and discussion," she says. "Let's run through his medical history."

"How long do you have?" I am trying to be funny, but I'm not funny. I shift into serious mode. I start with the night of his first seizure and work forward.

"Don't forget the time he had the seizure at Rainbow Foods," Tyler fills in details that I miss. The nurse jots something down. I wonder if she is logging the story or if she is noting that the five-year-old is the family historian.

Porter sits on the couch but he has a seizure and ends up on the floor. I get him on his side and it stops. Tyler explains it was a petite mal. She looks at the nurse. "A petite mal is a seizure." The nurse looks concerned and I don't know if it is for Porter, or for Tyler, or for the precariousness of the whole situation.

Half an hour later it is time for her to go. Porter is awake again and walking around the edge of the coffee table on wobbly legs. He spies her pen and leans in and grabs it. The nurse is kneeling on the ground, putting her clipboard in her cloth bag. It says something about the library association and I wonder about this briefly and then am distracted.

Porter walks up close, grabs her ponytail, and pulls with both hands. She grabs it above where he holds on to stop the pulling and it looks like they are caught in a tug-of-war.

"No Porter!" I say, but I say it too loud and Porter giggles the way he always does when someone seems excited. The neurologist says he can't differentiate between yelling angrily and excitement and that it all sounds like a basketball game to Porter. Finally, he lets go of her hair and claps.

"Good job, Porter," he says.

The nurse is still holding her head. I'm half-glad she saw his behavior and half-embarrassed. She begins to go down her checklist, asking whether he can do this or whether he can do that. The answer is no for every question she asks, no matter what it is.

She tries to get Porter to write a letter and he takes the pencil and tries to poke her eye. This time I am faster and I grab his arm, and she shuts her notebook and stands up to go.

One week later we get a call that we have qualified for the program. I ask how this happened—wondering about the years of waiting, but the administrator cuts in and tells me, "Especially tough cases go to the front of the line."

I don't know whether to feel happy or distressed that we are at the top of the list for disability severity. I choose to be happy and a week later we all are thrilled when our Personal Care Attendant (PCA) arrives for Porter.

Our PCA comes in the form of a twenty-seven-year-old ex-stripper and recovering addict named Jasmine. I know these things because she tells me her life story in our first five minutes together. This is our job interview and I hire her on the spot. Give me someone that's eager for the job and I'll take them. Heartbeat? Hired.

Jasmine isn't scared of seizures since she's seen people die before.

"Not a client," she clarifies, "an ex." This seems worthy of probing, but I don't.

We move on to her schedule. She is with us three nights a week from 3–8 p.m. The timing is good.

I feel like I just won the Powerball.

We adjust to the seizures, but not the side effects of the Depakote that's meant to control them. The good news is that the drug has not killed him. But it does cause behavioral issues—no form of discipline works. We start a new drug to treat the side effects of the drug to treat his seizures. I am glad that Jasmine sees this instantly when she comes with me to see Dr. Garrison that afternoon.

Porter spies the LEGO table and moves in like a heat-seeking missile. A minute later, he throws a block into the bassinette of a tiny baby.

"Don't throw that at the baby, Porter," I yell.

He laughs.

"You'll hurt the baby."

Hysterical laughter.

"I'll take the LEGOs away if you do that again." I hear the sternness in my voice. A LEGO lands in my lap. I scoop up all the blocks and take them away. Porter lies on his back and kicks the table.

The good parents look over. The good children look over. Jasmine files her nails.

Porter looks me in the eye and says, "You scare me." He says that a lot. He doesn't know what it means but he says it anyway. "You scare me, Mommy," he repeats. He usually says this when we are in public, surrounded by spectators. He sounds convincing, even to me.

I pick Porter up and carry him to the receptionist to see if we can hide in an exam room.

"Number three on the left," she says, glad to have us go. As I carry Porter, he kicks me.

"Stop it," I tell him.

"You scare me," he says again.

Jasmine chews her gum with a blank stare.

This continues as we leave the doctor's office. We have hit the point that total strangers give me parenting tips. A woman in the waiting room says I need to be firm. She raises her eyebrows to show me she's serious. I give her a look back that says, *I'm dropping the ball but I try.* I smile at the stranger. Porter kicks me.

We walk to our car, which is parked in the nearby Target parking lot. I set Porter down to unlock the door. He bolts to the other side of the car and starts laughing. I run one way and he runs the other. I chase him in a circle around my Toyota.

"Stop it," I say.

Laughter.

"Stop it, Porter."

More laughter. I get down on my hands and knees and look under the car. I see his legs, his Velcro tennis shoes by the back wheel. They light up every time he jumps. I crawl around the car on all fours to surprise him. A woman watches me and drives her shopping cart into a parked minivan. I grab Porter by the ankle and pull him. The woman is still watching me. I strap Porter into his seat.

She is mouthing something. "Ritalin," she says.

We get home and I hand Porter to Jasmine to talk with Brian in the kitchen.

We have Jasmine, but we lose Mary. She's decided to close her day care as her kids are in school and she feels she needs a new job. We scramble for a new option. There is one fewer issue we face in the sales pitch: Porter stopped using the breathing monitor when he turned one. Mary refers us to her church where the day care program has an opening for both our kids.

It is a sunny, active, loving place that advertises, "We love all differences." We'll see.

Porter's hyperactivity is manageable as long as the Depakote stops the seizures. But it doesn't stop them and the behavior gets worse. When Porter starts jumping off chairs, I learn a valuable lesson: Nothing gets blood out of carpet. It is stained that evening when Porter climbs on our desk chair to jump, but he has a seizure first and he hits the wooden edge on his way down. I am in the kitchen with Tyler when I hear the thud. I freeze and listen, hearing only the ticking of the kitchen clock as the second hand pulses around the dial. I run upstairs and find Porter on his side, arms clutched in the fetal position, tremors moving through his body. He is twisted and rigid and his hand grips a matchbox car. A red ring lines the carpet near his face. He is bleeding so much that the liquid pools and tiny bubbles appear along the edge. There is spatter on the wall he is pressed against, and I wonder what the cast-off pattern would tell a forensic detective.

I pull a pair of socks out of the laundry basket beside us to stop the flow. I scream for Tyler to scream for Brian. The seizures stop a minute later with a final shudder running through his body. The bleeding ebbs when I press hard enough. I pick him up and carry him downstairs, my arms red and smeared as I cradle him close. He is deadweight against my chest and his arms are outstretched, bumping the doorjamb as I carry him to the living room. The bleeding finally stops and Brian strokes his head when I set him on the couch. We don't say anything. He moves him into his lap and the bleeding resumes. It stains Brian's shorts and the couch. I run to the kitchen and grab a dish towel, and we hold it against Porter's head. We wait for more bleeding and we wait for more seizures, and when neither one happens I go upstairs and look at the scene.

There is a stain on the rug that stretches out in two circles, like a sideways number eight. Like the symbol for infinity:

looping and endless. I need to get rid of the blood and I scrub it with water and soap and it spreads farther and deeper into the carpet fibers. I scrub harder and start crying. I scrub even harder and it won't come out. I need to remove the evidence, but the evidence remains. I finally give in and put a towel over the spot the way a sheet is pulled up to hide the face of a dead person. We take Porter to the ER and his head is shaved across the back. They stitch the cut in two lines like a cross on the back of his skull.

We spend the next few days walking past the towel. We avert our eyes the way you do when you pass a fatal crash on the highway.

In the end, we replace the whole carpet.

I call my father to talk about what is happening. I ramble for five minutes without a breath.

"It sounds incredibly tough, sweetie," he says.

"I am fighting with Brian, the case is barely moving, and I feel like a horrible mother." I lay it all out on the line for him.

"You are a wonderful mother," he says, trying to reassure me.

"What makes that true is results, not words. I want an emotional lever to change how I feel."

"I bet you do."

"It kills me that I haven't found anything that helps Porter."

"I remember reading something once about how organisms develop and the fact that creatures don't struggle to evolve; they evolve due to struggle," he says. "Life is incredibly hard sometimes and it seems like the best we can do is learn and grow in the process. You are doing that. You've always been a fighter. You are resilient and you will get through this."

"The parenting rubber hit the road and I've careened off course. What about helping him get better?"

"Maybe the goal isn't to change him but to be with him in this struggle."

I think about these words. The gift my father has given me is being with me throughout this struggle. I need to be with Porter during his.

I hear Brian return from a late-night grocery run. Porter wouldn't sleep so he brought him to Rainbow. Now he slings Porter over a shoulder to bring him to bed. Porter hits his back and screams. Brian shuts the door behind him. He's singing a John Denver song to Porter. I stand in the hall for a few minutes, just listening.

11

Our new day care, Welcome Home, has an open house that they model after teacher-parent conferences.

Our teacher, Brianna, pulls out a folder. She talks quickly and taps her foot as if she's listening to music the rest of us can't hear. The teacher's notes are written in cursive and the space after Tyler's name is filled with exclamation points.

"She has such a curious mind! There are so many things she wants to learn about!" the woman says as we sit in tiny chairs around the kids' lunch table. "I wrote down Tyler's questions in class because, honestly, I wasn't able to answer a few of them!" The teacher pulls out a page and starts reading out loud.

"Here is what she asked. This is just last week! 'How is plastic made?,' 'Why are their unions?,' 'Why doesn't Jamaica have a real winter when the earth rotates halfway around every six months?,' and 'What do ants do with their larvae while they are working outside the nest?' That last one was a stumper. I told her I had to get back to her." The teacher smiles. "You must be doing something right at home!"

I am at a loss for words and reach for her notes to read over Tyler's questions. I want to savor this part of the conference since I know Porter's session will have a different kind of tone. I keep my own notes about his developmental milestones and I know his progress has stalled, even begun to slip backwards.

The conversation with Porter's teacher is short. In the *strengths* category she has written "accurate pouring," and we mainly discuss this. I assume this means sand on the playground. In the *developing* category, every box is checked. Below it is a page of notes. I see the phrase "trouble with transitions" written three times, and underlined.

It is time to go and we have trouble with transitions. Brian carries Porter out and I walk behind them, holding Tyler's hand. She doesn't mention larvae or unions, but she does skip as we walk to the car.

"At least Porter got one A," she says. I assume she is referring to his skilled pouring and I am surprised that she heard this. "They don't score him on the things that Porter is really good at. They should have other grades."

"Like what?" I ask.

"Porter never gets mad that he has seizures every day. That's an A. He never says, 'Why do I have to go to the hospital all the time!?' That's an A. And when I was crying the other day he came over and hugged me."

I squeeze Tyler's hand tighter. I see what she sees in Porter. And I see in her what she does not see in herself.

A traveling fair is in town and Tyler spots it as we drive past. She begs for us to go. It sounds like a good idea—to get out of the house, to have family time. We pack up the kids, as well as Porter's drugs, and walk to the park.

The air is thick and wet. People press past us. Kids are screaming, laughing, and crying. The merry-go-round melody circles us and Porter lies on the midway like a beached whale. Crowds do this to him. The neurologist says it's like circuit board overload. Porter refuses to stand up or move. Two people step on him. Brian picks him up then sets him down, and Porter runs to the Ferris wheel through the cordoned-off area under the steps. It is dark and greasy. It is a place where the bottom of a chair will hit you in the head if you stand there long enough. Brian pulls him out and carries him sideways under an arm.

"I want to ride the Ferris wheel," Tyler says.

We look at each other debating what to do. One person can take Porter home, but it isn't family time if you only have half a family. Brian offers to take Porter away. Tyler and I get on the Ferris wheel, and a man shuts the bar across our laps.

"The bar's loose so don't stand up," he says, grinning. His bottom teeth are gone and I smell alcohol on his breath. "It'll be real exciting if you do," he adds. I put an arm around Tyler and we sail up to the top, then stop, jerking in the breeze.

"That man smelled," Tyler says, "just like grandpa that time after he mowed the lawn and had a beer." A toothless morning drinker, this is the man in charge of our safety.

"He's probably sweaty from how hot it is," I reassure her.

"But Mom, his sweat smells like that. Grandpa let me smell the can and it was gross."

We stay at the fair all morning. It is easy with just Tyler.

The day after the fair we are at it again as a family, this time taking Porter to a park, hoping he will burn off his energy. I'm hoping it will burn off without his neurons firing randomly. As I watch Porter play, I sit by a woman and a boy in a wheelchair. Her child is strapped into the seat but is tilted to the side. I ask her about him and we start to talk. We cut right to the chase. We know the secret twin language you share with other parents like this.

"He was born with a number of things wrong with him and weighed only twenty pounds at age two. He can't eat so he has a feeding tube."

I look at her boy. He is slumped in a chair with just one eye open.

"Can he talk?" I ask.

"No. Sometimes he blinks to communicate."

This makes me think of what I've read of Jean-Dominique Bauby. He was the editor of *Elle* magazine until a massive stroke at the age of forty-three severed his brain stem from his spinal column. Following a three-week coma he woke paralyzed and mute, though his mind was untouched. His *locked-in syndrome* was described in his memoir, transcribed by a friend who translated eye blinks to letters in the alphabet.

The woman wants to know about Porter. He is squealing as he pours sand between buckets. I tell her about his brain damage. Then I tell her all of the things he loves, like blowing bubbles, his sister, and the sound of the vacuum as it whirs over the carpet. The woman and I sit and watch. We watch without saying anything.

She looks haggard. I can see in her what people see in me. I know why they ask me if I am tired. They aren't imagining it. Research has shown the link between psychological stress and biological age and the role cell division plays. Researchers found that blood cells from female caregivers of disabled children appeared to be ten years older than those of a matched group who did not have disabled children. The scientists evaluated the DNA of white blood cells because they play a key role in immunity.

They zeroed in on the telomere, which is the dangly end of every cell's chromosomes. Cells constantly divide and replicate themselves and the telomere shortens each time this happens. It's a lot like what happened to the quality of cassette tapes I made as a teenager that I copied from my friend's copies. The length of this telomere tip mirrors our biological age. This division is natural as we grow up or fight infection. A natural chemical called telomerase rebuilds the wispy tail. After a certain number of these events, the telomere eventually wears out and the cell commits a type of cell suicide to avoid becoming cancerous.

When the doctors compared the DNA of the caregivers and controls, they found that the longer women cared for disabled children, the shorter their telomeres. The chemical change agent telomerase was well below what is considered normal for women their age. The chronic effects of caring for these children were accelerating their aging in a biological sense.

When I get home from the park, I tell Brian about the woman's son. How he can't sit up or talk or eat—just blink that one eye.

"It really puts things in perspective about Porter," I say.

"At least with that kid's disabilities you could read a lot," he says back.

I talk to my mother on the phone and she is worried about my health. She probably senses my stubby telomeres. She also thinks Tyler is getting the short end of the stick. She worries the focus on Porter means we are all going downhill.

12

THREE AND A HALF YEARS

I'm thinking nonstop of Ritalin since the woman said it in the parking lot. I take Porter to the neurologist's office so we can crack the code on hyperactivity. We've always erred on the side of avoiding more medications. Now that seems quaint.

"I think he needs amphetamines," Jasmine says. She has a pharmacist-like knowledge of drugs that she picked up in narcotics anonymous. In the doctor's office Porter turns on the faucet and drops a piece of chalk down the drain. I put him on the exam table for a reflex check, and he jumps into the doctor's lap and knocks over his medical bag.

"He's quick," the doctor jokes.

"No, Porter," I scold him. Porter grabs a second piece of chalk and puts it in the drain. "No, Porter," I repeat.

The doctor signals him over. "Hey Porter, can you come over here and let me check your eyes?" he asks nicely. He is always nice.

Porter puts the chalk in his mouth. "No, Porter," I say again. I wonder if he thinks that his name is No Porter.

The doctor leans over and whispers, "It may be a good idea to try the Ritalin because hyperactivity can affect his self-esteem if he's always getting in trouble."

Porter puts the chalk in his diaper. I smile. I don't say no.

"It might," I say. I tell the doctor that I will discuss it with Brian.

As soon as I get home, I bring it up to Brian. He doesn't go for it. I launch into sell mode. "The doctor thinks it will help calm him down and then we won't have to say no so much. Porter will have better self-esteem." I realize that I am arguing about self-esteem and he doesn't even know his ABCs.

"I don't want him on more drugs," says Brian. "I don't think it is that bad."

I watch Porter put a toy car in his diaper. This is his latest routine—to hide things in his pants. I used to fish them out, but now I cut my losses.

"It is that bad," I shoot back, "and being the one home with him half-days every day, I think that I have a better idea about it."

"Why do you always bring up how much more time you spend with the kids?"

"I bring it up because it seems relevant to consider how much time we both actually take care of him."

"You're just being competitive," he replies.

I should stop, I think. *I can't stop*. "If saying I spend more time with him when I actually do spend more time is competitive then, yes, I am competitive. I want to try Ritalin because maybe it will help."

Brian doesn't respond.

I win the argument but I lose anyway because when we try the Ritalin, it has no effect on Porter.

My work at the university is divided between the neurology clinic and field research in area nursing homes. In both settings, my clients have dementia and mental illness. This week I am sitting in a locked Alzheimer's unit in Roseville. I go to the institution to observe the clients and see how often they are physically aggressive with the staff. It's pretty often. The patients are confused about where they are and who they are.

One man named Ernest tells me about weekends he spends at home on his farm. It takes three weeks before I realize that he never leaves the ward and the only farm he's visited is at the Minnesota Zoo. Today he is angry. His pants are hiked to his chest and he looks like a sleep-deprived Captain Kangaroo. He disappears back out of sight and I hear him knock loudly on something.

"*Nurse!*" he yells. "Anybody work around here?"

"Can I help you Ernest?" a woman's voice asks.

"I'm glad I'm back here because I'm having some problems when I go home on the weekends," he says. "I know I'm not supposed to swear but the food there was really shitty. Oops. Sorry. I said I wouldn't cuss. We just worked on that in my anger therapy, but if you don't do something, I'm going to be really pissed and tell Dr. Drake. Oops. I said I wouldn't threaten anyone—but I'm fucking mad."

"Ernest . . ." she says, her tone is unhappy.

Ernest stops talking and there is silence once more. He prowls the hall, then plops down next to me on the couch. "Nobody gives you a straight story. You know what I mean?" he asks me. I know what he means.

Ernest is pacing again a few feet away. He leans on the medication counter and yells, "I didn't eat all weekend because the food was so shitty." When no one answers, he continues, "I'm starving to death." I glance at the calendar with the giant shiny sun hanging over the desk in front of us.

As I get up to go back to the office, I hear Ernest scream, "Hey nurse, do you want to go out to dinner?"

I find Melinda, the woman I am here to see. It is time for her monthly neuropsychological testing we are doing as part of a double-blind, placebo-controlled study of antipsychotic medication and Alzheimer's patients. This is my dissertation study.

I am sitting in a windowless room behind the nurses' station. The tests I give gauge memory and coherence; and I'm having trouble getting her to answer my questions.

"Can you write out a sentence for me?" I'm administering a test called the mini–mental state examination and am moving through a series of questions one by one. At the moment I am asking her to identify common objects and I hold up a pencil. Melinda stares at it like she's never seen one.

"Can you write out a sentence for me?" I ask again.

She grabs the pencil and scribbles fast. "This one's for you," and she hands it to me. The words "SHUT UP!" are scrawled in capitals.

"I have something far more important to discuss," she says. I put the test down. Sometimes the best thing I can do is listen.

"What's that?" I ask.

"It's a scam. They write all these wonderful things about saving the animals, but it's really just a pyramid scheme." She pulls a piece of paper out of her bag and shakes it. I feel sorry for Melinda as well as her husband, who is pretending to read a book behind her.

"What are you talking about Melinda?"

"This adopt-an-endangered-monkey B.S.," she says. "Jane Goodall writes me a letter and says I can adopt a monkey—you know, just send in your money and he'll be yours—but it's a fraud. No monkey, no nothing."

"Are you sure you understood what it said?"

Melinda shakes her head and says, "Of course I did. I've studied those little hairballs forever. You know they can talk now—they taught them sign language and they communicate perfectly. They're tricky little devils though. Jane Goodall spends all her life in the forest teaching one of them to speak and the first thing out of his mouth is a swear word. It really makes me wonder how my tax dollars are being spent."

"What did you sign up for Melinda?"

"This!" She holds the magazine page out and shakes it again. "Jane *said* you send fifty dollars a month and you adopt it, so I sent my cash, right to the P.O. Box here, and nothing—no monkey," she tells me, emphasizing the fact that there is no monkey.

I try to reason with her. This is my other bad habit. "It actually says that you send the money and it supports research. You don't actually adopt the animal. Your money goes towards conservation."

"Riiiight, that's what it says. I'm onto Goodall's little game, and I'm not going to go quietly about this, either. Let's see if Sigourney Weaver still wants to play her in the sequel when I'm done with her."

I put down the test. *Anger is a moral response.* "I'm sorry that happened," I say to her.

Melinda puts the paper away and stands up. She takes a deep breath and says, "I think it's time to go home and take care of my babies." Melinda's husband stands up. He is eighty years old. She is seventy-four. He grabs his cane and pauses a foot behind Melinda.

"She's having a bad day," he says. "We'll see you next week." I watch them leave the waiting area, holding hands.

It crosses my mind that her husband never gets angry that he deals with this every day. If Tyler were grading him, he'd get an A.

13

Porter developed encephalopathy within twelve hours of his DPT and is a specified table injury. When we leave the appointment with Katherine and hear that the case will soon be done and the government will soon be responding to our petition in thirty days, Brian and I are holding hands, almost skipping. I wonder why the case has taken this long, but it isn't helpful asking why. When the tire blows you fix it; you don't sit on the side of the road wondering why it's flat.

I call my parents. I call my best friend Nina. I am animated and upbeat since we are two months from the finish line. This isn't simply my typical hypomanic enthusiasm; I know what the results will be! Studies have found that people like a story better when they know the ending. It removes the cognitive load of having to decipher every twist and turn as it unfolds. You can reserve that strength or brainpower for the process. I can see the finish line.

Nicholas Christenfeld and Jonathan Leavitt of UC San Diego confirmed this finding empirically when they found that subjects preferred reading classic short stories prefaced by a paragraph that provided a spoiler alert for the ending.[14]

After all the frowns and condescending comments from health professionals and others in the world, there is vindication in knowing we are not crazy. It is a contradiction in itself to say that vaccines are unequivocally safe while a Federal Court exists to adjudicate the injuries and death.

To deny vaccine problems isn't far-fetched, it's a part of human nature. We seek to avoid the discord created by a discrepancy between what we believe and publically advocate for, and the facts. To promote an unflinching safety in vaccines while meeting a brain-damaged child generates something called cognitive dissonance. When this arises, our tendency is to reject conflicting evidence and stick to our beliefs. It doesn't matter that we tell our pediatrician about the vaccine court, which she never knew existed. Or that the ER physician told her that Porter's encephalopathy was caused by the vaccine. Or that our neurologist wrote a letter of support. Or that we have a table injury. No matter what conflicting data we present, she says again, "Vaccines never cause harm."

In an attempt to help Porter with his repetitive language, we sign him up for speech therapy but the speech therapist says she can't test him, that we need another specialist—one that treats "his kind of problem." Whatever that is.

I am not dissuaded. There are other specialists and I want to try all of them. If Porter had cancer, we'd be using shark cartilage by now. But Brian is tired of all the cures—Brian is tired all the time. We fight. We try not to fight. We fight about what our fighting means.

In the middle of this, Tyler tries to get our attention. She tells me one afternoon, "I want to ride in an ambulance, too; then you could visit me in the hospital."

14 Jonathan D. Leavitt and Nicholas J.S. Christenfeld, "Story Spoilers Don't Spoil Stories." *Psychological Science*, 2011. doi:10.1177/0956797611417007.

Soon after, she starts to act out. She spits and hits me at bedtime and announces she will not go to sleep. She says she will wait to sleep until we get up later with Porter's next seizure. I carry her back to her room with her legs in the air.

When I finally go to bed, Brian stirs and says, "I'm wide awake. I've been backlogged on sleep for two years."

"You'll feel better once we get up."

"You never sound sympathetic to how I am doing." He turns his back to me. I don't say anything because he's right. I don't feel sympathetic.

Brian, Tyler, and I are all trying to manage our family life while everyone is a casualty. In one of my graduate courses we read about the Post-Traumatic Stress ailing at least one out of six family members of a severely ill child. Nancy Kassam-Adams has a PhD and directs the center for Pediatric Traumatic Stress at the Children's Hospital in Philadelphia. She says that the trickiest part is maintaining self-care. It's common to lapse into feelings of hopelessness when our parental default to protect our children doesn't work.

The depression and anxiety we feel is referred to as "learned helplessness." I know about this phenomenon from my studies, as it is seminal in psychology. The research dates back to the 1960s when it was first discovered. One of the professors in my department was an original researcher on the data. Over the years it has been applied to everything from trauma and illness to people in war zones. It strikes me that our household hits all categories.

The initial data went something like this: Dr. Martin Seligman conducted research with dogs in which they were held in cages with metal floors. A tone sounded and a shock occurred and they quickly learned to jump out over a small wall to escape the pain.

In the next condition there was no way to get free. When the animals were restrained in the cages they learned that no matter what they did, they could not get away from the shock. They still heard the tone, but after struggling to get loose, they simply lay on the floor, whimpering until the shock subsided. This seems predictable, but what they found in the next phase of experimentation was not.

In the third condition, the same dogs were freed from restraint and the warning tone sounded again. Instead of jumping out of the cage, the animals cowered and cried despite the fact that they were no longer trapped. The dogs had learned to be helpless. This research quickly generalized to what happens to humans when faced with insurmountable challenge. When the circumstances ensue despite all efforts, most humans simply give in and no longer try to escape.

I could see the pull to lie down and whimper. But good mothers don't do that, good mothers find a way to help their children jump over the wall to escape.

During each appointment our pediatrician, Dr. Amit, says that Porter is about to catch up. He has missed every developmental milestone since his last birthday. In fact, he's going backwards. I listen for new information, but nothing ever comes. I keep asking about autism but I am told that it is too soon to diagnose. But now that Porter is three years old, she changes her tune.

"It's possible he has autism," the doctor says the next time we see her.

"You scare me," Porter replies.

The doctor pauses. "What scares you?" She is looking at me. Then Porter. Then me. "What scares you, Porter?" she asks again.

"I like Pocahontas," he replies.

She's not giving up. "Are you scared?"

Porter looks the other way. "Tigger's stuck in a tree."

The doctor is back to business.

"We'll set you up for some testing. I get the sense that he may have a developmental delay."

I get the sense that it's time to leave, since Porter has a handful of tongue depressors stuck down his pants.

The neuropsychologist works at Courage Center. He's in a room above the one for my support group and we go there a week after the discussion with our pediatrician. His office is a swirl of books and papers, there's a tripod with a camera in the corner and a bowl of M&Ms on his desk.

"What is the candy for?" I wonder how it fits into psychometrics.

"Occasionally I have parents that think the issue is a hearing problem versus intentional. I have devised a very scientific way to determine the difference."

"You bribe them?" I like the doctor more every minute.

"This is a trick I didn't learn at Harvard. I had a boy last week that was a bundle of energy and never followed instructions. The parents thought he was hard of hearing. I told them I could answer that without any auditory exam." Dr. Cohen smiles and it's obvious he likes his job. "The boy was bouncing all over the place and wouldn't sit down when his mother asked him to. As he stood with his back to us I whispered, 'Do you want to clean up your room?' and he didn't budge. Then I whispered, 'Do you want some M&Ms?' And he whirled around—definitely not a hearing problem!"

"Great idea." I am impressed.

"I'm not necessarily endorsing bribery," he adds.

Dr. Cohen grabs his binder and proceeds to explain the testing process. We are breaking up the testing between a Friday and the following Monday since six hours of testing would be quite a stretch.

Dr. Cohen sits across from Porter at a tiny table with a puzzle on top of it. Porter takes the pieces and stacks them in a pile. The doctor removes each piece from the stack to show Porter how they fit together. I stick around for the first test to make sure things are okay. As I leave the room, I see Porter has matched each piece.

I walk downstairs to the heated therapy pool. There's a class in session to teach children with disabilities to swim. A boy with cerebral palsy walks along the edge, one step up, one step down. The parents are on the side in chairs cheering.

When I retrieve Porter at the end of the day, I'm pleased to see that Dr. Cohen is smiling. I do this often: gauge people's body language after they spend time with my son to see if they are ready to kill him.

Porter is at the table, apparently back to stacking puzzle pieces in a pile. Dr. Cohen has a folder of notes and tells me we'll finish the tests on Monday.

"Any initial thoughts?" I ask. This is the moment of truth, the time we'll find out the official label that describes our life. Brian is wary of pinning a name on what Porter has since it might follow him in school. I, on the other hand, am eager to diagnose. I am hoping this will lead to a battalion of therapists, armed with the right treatment to get Porter back to normal.

"I only have preliminary tests, but it is interesting," he says. *Interesting* is a Minnesota word that doesn't mean fascinating, but iffy. Midwesterners have a special language for negative things that allows them to talk without ever sounding mean.

"Channel your New York side, Dr. Cohen," I tell him. "Be blunt."

"Some of his scores are very low. His speech tests are in the second percentile. His receptive language is nonexistent," he says to me.

My reaction to this is mixed: 25 percent validated and 75 percent panicked. It strikes me that the number of words Porter has mastered is not paying off. The words need to mean something to count.

"There is also good news," he continues. I worry that he is backing away from the moment, trying to buffer the facts with happy news. Dr. Cohen shuffles through his stack and pulls out one test. "He is actually above average on his spatial ability. Such uneven abilities are definitely brain injury. That is my formal diagnosis after the testing."

My mind goes back to our second trip to the hospital when we realized the seizure was not a fluke. The words of the ER doctor pop into my head and I think about the fact that what we see—the perseverating, the flapping, the knack for puzzles—is an outgrowth of Porter's neurological problems. This is what happens when a baby's brain is damaged right out of the chute. Bad things follow and now we have a test that proves it.

I ask Dr. Cohen to go back to what he said about Porter's language problems relating directly to his behavior problems.

"Kids learn to calm themselves down when they can talk to themselves and say soothing things. Without the words to think that things will be okay, the problems tend to ensue," Dr. Cohen explains.

"So what if they can't ever talk to themselves?"

Dr. Cohen looks back and puts his binder down. "It can take a while before the tantrums work themselves out."

My mind races. No language equals permanent tantrums, equals Porter in prison. This sounds like a catastrophe so I struggle to redirect my thoughts to something more positive. But it's not positive. No matter how many ways I imagine our family life, it never leads to Disneyland. No matter how I try to reconfigure what Dr. Cohen has said, there is no way Porter's problems equal normal life.

"The results as to his future potential are not the most optimistic," he admits.

All I think is, *More bad news.*

"Formal education is highly unlikely," he continues. *Grade school dropout.*

"I don't see a professional job," he forces out. *Jail.*

"Just spit it out," I prompt.

"He will be in a sheltered workshop in the best scenario," he concludes. A shiver snakes down my back. I know all about sheltered workshops from my work with people with mental disabilities. In fact, I've spent whole weekends supervising my clients at Opportunities Unlimited. Images of OU leaps to mind: long tables filled with stacked crates, people yelling, people wearing helmets, someone wandering off to the wrong room, tall ceilings, manicured walkways, cigarette smoke, a handicap cab waiting outside. As soon as I leave the office, I call Brian to tell him this news. "I don't believe it," he says quickly.

Not surprisingly, when Tyler begins Montessori school, we get a different developmental story about her. "Yesterday I heard her talking to another five-year-old," her teacher says, "and she was telling the other girl that there wasn't enough blocks to build a tower. Tyler said, 'They've run out of LEGOs, so you'll have to improvise.' Seriously, she said, 'improvise.' Wow, you are raising smart kids!"

I want to correct her: We are raising a smart *kid.* She doesn't know Porter and doesn't realize there is no *s* on the end of the word *kid* in that sentence.

The problem is our smart kid doesn't want to go to bed at night. Each evening the same thing happens: Tyler negotiates to stay up, then screams, and then announces she will never rest. I know that she needs attention and I know that I should be tolerant. This works until 11:00 p.m. when I am exhausted and all reasoning fails so I find myself dragging her by an arm and a leg back into her bed.

She spits and hits when I get her there, and I see myself in her bedroom mirror and wonder who that woman is. We stop fighting and she climbs into bed between her father and me.

A few minutes later I whisper to Brian, "Can you sleep with all of us in here?" Tyler rolls over. "Definitely," she says.

We are all asleep in less than a minute. She sleeps in our bed with us every night until we no longer sleep together.

14

FOUR YEARS

That summer, we take one last stand for normalcy. Two stands, really—one by plane and one by car. Each is a disaster. The flight comes first. My sisters want us to visit California. I know they mean well. These trips and the family time always sound good in theory, minus the flying. I head out with my children, alone, so I can leave a few days early, and Brian can join us for the weekend. I like the idea of strapping Porter into his booster on the plane and having him restrained for several hours. I imagine finishing a novel and sipping Diet Coke. I like the idea until we have a mechanical problem and the plane is stranded next to the gate. The bridge is pulled away and there is no escape unless you jump. It's not long before I want to jump.

One hour turns into two hours, and then two turns into four. The Diet Coke spills. The book slides under the seat. I have a hyperactive boy next to me who no longer wants to be on the airplane.

"We are *all done with this*!" he says, because that's what he tells you when the jig is up.

"I think Porter wants to get off the plane," Tyler says.

"We can't get off the plane," I remind her. Porter grabs his bag of crackers and throws it across the aisle and it hits a passenger. He is an old man who wears an oxygen mask. Porter arches his back and kicks the seat in front of him. I grab his feet and hold them, hunched over and talking to him sideways in a stern whisper.

"We are all done with this," Porter repeats.

The woman next to me nods and I assume it is because she's glad I'm taking charge. I make a shushing sound and tell Porter to stop. He is unmoved. The passengers are annoyed and Porter is restless. I want to kick my seat. Instead, I try signing his favorite song, "Country Roads," since he's fixated on John Denver and listens to him around the clock. Porter put his hand over my mouth to stop me. I whisper again, trying to sound firm for the other passengers who may or may not want to kill us.

The pilot comes on over the loudspeaker. "Good news! Things are settled and we're second in line to take off." This would have been good news a few hours ago, but now it is bad news. Porter unbuckles his belt and runs towards the cockpit. The old man grabs his leg, then makes a funny face and Porter laughs.

I scoop him up and the flight attendant says into the microphone, "We can't move until everyone stays in their seats." I give a little wave to her and strap Porter in next to me.

Porter arches and says, "Don't hurt people!" The woman beside me looks worried, but says nothing and goes back to her John Grisham. I'm touched that she thinks I am abusing my son but doesn't report me to the pilot.

The food is gone and all bets are off.

As I restrain him, the old man in the mask tosses the bag of crackers back to Porter and winks at him. I want to hug the old man. When the flight finally starts, we are allowed to get up and head to the back. We spend the next two hours in the bathroom flushing the toilet. It whooshes each time and Porter claps and flaps. We stay like this and no one knocks. The other passengers are pleased we are gone. They share one toilet since I'm almost positive no one wants the autistic kid back in the middle of the plane.

As we lower again, a baby behind us starts to wail and heads snap around to see if it is us. Typically we are the problem and I savor the experience of not being the center of attention. We circle around and circle again. The pilot comes onto the loud speaker.

"Folks, you've probably noticed we're circling. I don't want anyone to worry, but the instruments are saying there is a potential issue with our landing gear. I'm fairly sure it's an error, but out of an abundance of caution we're going to have some emergency vehicles out by the landing. Again, I believe this is not serious, but you may see some fire trucks." The plane is silent. The woman next to me takes a deep breath.

Porter claps his hands and screams, "Woohoo! Fire trucks!"

The flight home is on time, but equally painful. No more planes.

Unwilling to give up entirely on vacations, we try one more time that summer and take a road trip to the Black Hills of South Dakota. We drive across the plains, the scene outside the car is flat and treeless. We crack the windows and a hot breeze swirls through the windows. Miles and hours elapse without any buildings.

The car in front of us has a sticker that reads I BRAKE FOR WALL DRUG, and we too brake for Wall Drug, parking on a dusty road outside a fake saloon. There's a horse hitch but no horses and a studio where you can dress up in old-fashioned clothing. I step out of the car and hot air hits my face. Dirt swirls around and gets in my teeth. Porter slaps the front of his car seat rhythmically and the door handle burns my fingers when I reach over to get Tyler. Brian picks up Porter and we wind through the closest building, looking at fake spiders and grabbing handfuls of pink penny candy. We walk through the connecting rooms: one a studio, one a restaurant, one filled with bumper stickers of South Dakota.

Brian and I have driven to the Black Hills most years since we married. This place calms me. I love the shooting gallery and animals to climb on. It's a place we always stop. Tyler grabs Porter's hand and leads him to the climbing structure ringed by benches. She knows exactly where to go and he will follow her anywhere. I sit to watch them. Tyler scrambles to the top of a ladder and Porter sits on the ground pouring sand from hand to hand. Tyler waves. Porter flaps. I hold Brian's hand and lean into his neck. We are a normal family. We play, we eat, and we are back on the road.

I savor this moment. I love watching my children playing normally in front of me and want to shut one eye to burn the image into my brain. I am relieved and I am calm. Everything is going to be all right.

The sign says KOA KAMPGROUND and has an arrow that points to the campsite. We pull into the drive way, register at the A-shaped office, get a map that shows our site with an X, and get back in the car to drive over there. The RVs are in one area and the tents in the other and the two sides are identical. It is flat and dusty and there are wooden picnic benches next to each fire pit. I hold Brian's hand and take a deep breath. The air smells like trees. Tyler and Porter are handing puzzle pieces back and forth as they sit in their car seats in the row behind us. Country music wafts over a loudspeaker and we pass little cabins with shingling around the roofs. A chain-link fence surrounds the property, and in the distance you can see Mount Rushmore.

We turn into the campsite, drive under a swaying sign that reads BADLANDS, unpack the minivan, and take the kids to the pool shaped like a kidney. Families sit in plastic chairs drinking beer and playing music. Two men sit a few feet away talking. The old man looks like the young man.

"You know you're getting up there when you think the mothers are better looking than the daughters." This comes from the father wearing a "Buy American" cap. He has the bulge of tobacco in his cheek and leans back. "Take those Judd sisters. Naomi's the good-looking one."

The woman next to me pours baby oil on her legs and shuts her eyes to the sun. She doesn't watch her children because they are older or don't have seizures or because she doesn't know that bad things can happen. The man in a Budweiser shirt screams at his son. His son splashes again and the man screams again. Porter jumps in the pool and swims to the side. He's never had a lesson but can dog paddle his way for miles. Brian tosses Tyler off his shoulders. She laughs hysterically and frog kicks over for more. She climbs back up and he throws her again.

Porter is sitting on the steps next to them in water up to his neck. He is grinning. Each time Tyler looks at him, Porter giggles incessantly and flaps his arms at her. Porter reminds me of a study I read about elephants. When they see each other after a time away, they flap their ears and stamp their feet to let the others know they are excited. Every time his sister gazes in his direction, Porter flaps his arms and kicks his feet.

"How are you, Porter?" she asks, and waves.

Porter responds, "How are you, Porter?" *Flap-flap-flap.*

Porter doesn't answer questions, he only repeats things. But Tyler is his Mowgli: She's learned the code and can talk to him in his secret language. I look away at the hills and see the dark splotches of pines and shut my eyes just for a minute. When I open them again Porter is gone.

He is face down a few inches below the surface. He is in the position my camp counselor called "the dead man's float." His arms are outstretched as if praying and undulate in the currents of the water filter. Someone should do something. My body reacts and I stand up so fast my chair topples over. The woman who's next to me gets up too fast and she slips as she stands and clutches at a table.

We pull him out and set him on the side of the pool. I can't tell if he has swallowed water. We turn him on his side and he jerks. The other parents stand, beers in hand, frozen in place, staring at us. Porter swallowed water and it gurgles out, pink from the candy. His eyes are locked. I can only see whites. I am shivering. It's hot outside but the wind whips at my face. I get on my knees to be closer to him. My son gurgles and twitches. I am cold, on my knees, and begging, silently: *This is not happening. It can't be happening.* I turn him on his side to see if he is breathing. I am wondering if he will die. My hands move on their own, somehow they know what to do.

The pool is empty now and an inflated crocodile bobs in the wind and bumps against the side of it. I am wondering about what the other parents think; I don't want to but I do anyway. My hands continue to hold Porter on his side and after two minutes the shaking stops. He takes a gulp of air. His cheek is streaked pink and sticky, and he lets a breath out.

A man from the campground appears, panting and bends over us. "I called 9-1-1," he says and his breath smells like onions. Then he turns to the onlookers like a cop on TV and says, "Step back, there's nothing to see." There is something to see, so no one steps back.

Three hours ago we were in Wall Drug and our weekend and future lay ahead. Now it is gone. Our night will be spent at a hospital and the weekend is over and our future is blank. I am holding Porter and his head swings to the side. I'm thinking about our vacation even though I don't want to. I hear the siren. The screaming man waves them over to the pool with a cigarette in his hand. He takes charge and holds the kids back with his other arm. I can't look at the parents and I can't look at my husband. I demanded this vacation and now it is a wreck.

When the paramedics kneel next to Porter, I stare at the ground. I stare at my son. The stretcher is white and they strap him to it. The buckles, meant for adults, slip over his body. He doesn't twitch because the seizure is done. The pool is empty because the swimming is done. The families stare and my fingers touch Porter's foot and I want to hold Brian's hand but I don't. My son's eyes are shut, but he is breathing and I wipe the streaks off his face with the edge of my towel.

I look at Brian. It's as if there is a sliding glass door separating my husband from me. I can see him but I can't touch him. I am terrified. He is terrified. But, there is no tether that links us in this fear. It takes every drop of energy to contain my terror and I have nothing left to comfort him with. The same well of strength I tap to survive is the one we both need to offer something to the other. I want to reach out but I can't. He wants to help me, but he can't. Surviving this moment to survive the next moment drains anything left inside me.

I walk barefoot across the parking lot and the rocks cut my feet and I am glad. I want to feel pain because I want to feel something. I stand next to the ambulance. I stare in the windows and I look for my eyes in the reflection. I try to see why I did this, since nothing makes sense. The woman paramedic has short spiky hair and leans in the front seat to talk on a radio. She looks like a man but acts like a woman, and her voice is soft and I start to cry. She brushes Porter's head and I clutch his foot, and we ride to the hospital like that, each of us holding on to part of his body. I cry and she pats my leg and she comforts us both, but there is nothing to do.

The hospital in Rapid City is boxy and beige. It looks like all the other hospitals. There is a helipad in front and towers behind it that appear to be part of an apartment building. There is a view from the window, but there aren't any windows where Porter now sleeps attached to three tubes.

"Seizures don't hurt people," the doctor says when he comes in the room and sits across from me. He is wearing blue scrubs and looks tired. His hair is blond and his eyes are blue.

"Except when they're underwater and you drown." I sound angry because no matter how hard I try, I can't make things better.

"He didn't drown," the doctor says.

"He didn't drown," I repeat.

We wait it out: the postictal phase of the seizure in which he sleeps for days, the Valium hangover, the watching to see if he starts up again. I walk to the main doors at 2:00 a.m. to stand outside and look at the Black Hills. The mountains are the same and the hospital is the same, but I am not the same.

We leave the next morning in our minivan. We are back on the road. There are signs for Wall Drug, and Tyler says, "Can we climb on the jackalope?" She is remembering the plastic rabbit that sits by the entrance. It has antlers and crouches in the grass.

"We're driving home," I tell her.

"Why?"

"Why?" Porter echoes. It strikes me that Tyler doesn't realize our vacation is over.

"We need to get home."

"Okay," she says and frowns.

"Okay," Porter echoes.

We drive past the exits. Past the signs that say Glad You Made It! I am glad we made it. We get home and unpack the car, put Porter in his bed, and take Tyler to her room.

I check on them before I sleep and I find them in Porter's bed together. Tyler has her arm around her brother and they are sleeping curled in a spoon.

15

In my support group, I learn about a way to feed your child that keeps him seizure-free and off medication. The meeting starts and Julie jumps up and claps her hands like a cheerleader, "Ketogenic Diet!" she shouts at us. All the other women take a breath and give a neutral look they've perfected in the last four meetings. Julie isn't dissuaded. She rolls the TV out of the corner and pops a video in.

"I can't wait to show you this!" she exclaims and she claps again. I clap back automatically. She smiles at me and mouths *thank you.*

She stands in front of the group and says, "It's a clip from *20/20* profiling a doctor who uses high-fat meals to stop epilepsy!" Silence. "No more fruits and veggies—it's time for saturated fat!" She grins and I wonder how this will make all the fat kids skinny. I wonder if that bothers her since that is her mission.

The video shows a doctor who says we need to feed our kids enticing dishes made of mayonnaise and whipping cream. Eating fat around the clock causes ketosis, in which the body begins to burn its own muscle. Maybe the diet stabilizes the energy level in the brain or maybe it calms the neurons themselves. Either way, the doctor says ketosis stops seizures in the majority of people.

Julie is in sell mode now. "It isn't crazy, you guys. The Bible even talks about it!"

MJ gives her a look. "I think I missed that—which verse talks about the Ketogenic Diet?"

"Don't tease, MJ! This is serious business! Read Mark, chapter nine! Jesus tells a dad that he can stop his son's seizures with fasting and prayer. It's right in there—sometimes science isn't so current!" Julie twirls around and smiles. "It's right there," she says again. "I don't know how you get a better endorsement than Jesus!"

The primary driver of the Ketogenic Diet is the restriction of carbohydrates. This is easy in theory but brutal in practice. The diet is tricky, and getting the portions wrong throws everything off. I have to weigh the food and get it just right; the dietician warns me in our training about the dangers of one extra peanut. She says the key is to get an accurate metric scale, so I head off to the store. Walking into Walmart, I find a heavyset man near the pet aisle in a tight sweatshirt with a loon on it and a saying that reads, "All roads lead to Minnesota."

"I need help finding a scale, something that is precise and metric," I say, asking him for assistance.

He stands straighter and hikes his pants up. "We've got a good one that weighs to the half-ounce. Which Jenny Craig program do you go to?"

"None. I need a scale that weighs in grams," I explain.

"Grams?"

"Quarter grams, half grams, and grams," I say. "Do you have that?"

"I see." And he steps backwards. It is apparent from his expression that he has lost interest in going to weight-loss meetings altogether.

"Do you have one?"

"I see," he says again. And in that moment I see, too, that the man with the loon stretched across his chest is feeling superior.

"It has to be metric. It's for a special diet," I tell him, by way of explanation.

"*Sure* it does. I've got your number, sister."

"Excuse me?" I say to him.

"We're not *that* kind of store, and we cater to a *different* customer, if you catch my drift." I start to say something back, but before I can, he dismisses me by bending over a shelf to restock kitty litter, his Fruit of the Loom tag in full view.

A few days later we are poised to get started. It takes anywhere from two to seven days to get into ketosis and the launch begins fast. The plan is also called the long-chain triglyceride diet, as it has a fat to protein/carbohydrate ratio of 4:1. We start the fast in the hospital since the beginning requires medical supervision. Vitamin D, folic acid, iron, and calcium are handwritten on the board to compensate for the diet that misses most food groups.

The fasting starts at dinnertime on a Monday. A television is wheeled into his room with a stack of videos piled up on the cart.

"Of course we ask that the family doesn't eat in front of him," the nurse says as we settle into the room. "Not even gum." This seems simple enough until I remember how frequently I eat. I learned this when I took a medication a year before and was told to ingest it on an empty stomach. The only time this occurred was first thing in the morning if I was really on the ball. As a runner, I am continually hungry. Porter is continually hungry, too.

Now we sit together in his hospital bed watching Pooh videos as I try to distract him. Every few minutes he touches my arm and asks, "Bagel?"

The quickest route to ketosis entails vigorous exercise on an empty stomach while water is restricted. It is 3:00 p.m. and my son is lethargic and starving and not in the mood for push-ups. At 5:00 p.m., he is surly and famished.

"Don't hurt people!" he screams, until the nurse closes his door.

"Let's watch a video," I suggest.

He hits me. Then he puts his hands on my face and turns it to look at him. "Hungry," he says. I hug him and he wriggles free. Then he lies face down and cries in the bed.

At dinnertime the fast is over. His tray arrives and looks promising until we pull off the cover and see three melon ball–sized servings of butter. There is whipping cream in a small paper cup, like the kind you find in the bathroom. Porter dives in and finishes it in no time. He wipes the cream off his face with the back of his hand and licks the cup until it is dry.

"More?" he asks.

He looks at me and grabs my face again. This time I lie down and cry.

On the second night we get to go home. We feed Porter mayonnaise and butter and sneak into the other room to have bread. It's as if we've developed eating disorders simultaneously: We can only eat in secret. I weigh his portions and dole out the fat and study his body language for the hint of a tremor. A week passes without a seizure. We are out of the woods, so it is worth it.

The television is evil since every ten minutes an ad comes on that pitches non-sanctioned food content. We only watch videos, but even these have food scenes and Porter crawls close to the screen when the animated characters eat.

"Pizza?" he asks when I hand him some butter.

"This is your lunch!" I reply in a singsong voice.

I hear Tyler behind me in the pantry rustling through a bag. She is a closet eater now, since we've told her not to have non-diet foods in sight of her brother.

"Juice?" he says. "Tyler, *juice!*"

Tyler appears looking sheepish. She holds something behind her back.

"Sorry, Porter," she says. "Mom says all you can eat is mayonnaise." When I turn around she whispers to him, "I don't know why!"

We stick to the diet because the diet works. It works because he doesn't have seizures, but it doesn't work if you want to be a functional family. We all adjust any way we can. I know from my psychology classes that our coping strategies are set up in the early years; some people win the sweepstakes and are comforted by their mothers. This training was missing from my childhood, but I want to do it differently now with my own family. I want Tyler and Porter to know that no matter how hard things seem, they can lean on people close to them.

In one of my graduate classes I came across the research done by Harry Harlow on childhood attachment and the way it colors our adult behavior. He researched primates and his baby rhesus monkeys were separated at birth from their mothers and nursed by metal dolls. They'd drink their milk, and then would sit in the corner sucking their thumbs. They had a self-sufficiency that I related to.

"The monkeys learned to console themselves when they were anxious," he wrote.[15] Some of these babies were lucky: They had playtime with other monkeys and learned to lean on friends when the going was tough. It is easy to picture which group I'd be in: the self-sufficient category, preferring thumb sucking or vodka instead of turning to others.

But I wasn't totally alone. Long before I discovered vodka, I started to pray. I remember the first time I did it, as a ten-year-old whispering so no one would know. When my mother first was feeling "sick" I began to talk to God, telling God little

15 Harry F. Harlow and Stephen J. Suomi, "Social Recovery by Isolation-Reared Monkeys." *Proceedings of the National Academy of Sciences of the United States of America* 68, no. 7 (1971): 1534–538.

stories about what was happening. In those moments I felt peace and warm arms around me during the middle of my talk. I knew it was God reaching down and giving me a squeeze to say things were fine.

I shut my eyes now, curling into my bed to tell God my story. I imagine him talking to me in a voice like the father in *The Sound of Music*: caring, sensitive, and reassuring that I will make it over the snowy Alps to freedom. Even if he can't get us over the Alps, he is at least here to let us know we are not alone in the snow.

But the diet works. We are moving over the Alps.

On the second week of the eating plan, Porter spends his days lying on the living room floor fingering the edge of his blanket. He hits my hand when I approach him with butter. The other options aren't much better: heavy whipping cream, canola oil, and mayonnaise. I need to find artful ways to combine these. I break down and call Julie for advice.

"High five for you!" she says, when she hears we are trying the diet. "You've been keto-fied!" She tells me that she will bring her "keto recipes" to the next meeting, and she does. The top card reads, "The Fat Bomb." This has potential. It's a cheesecake that you eat for dinner. I shove the cards into my purse and pull them out that night to start cooking.

Tucked amongst the cards is a note from Julie covered in hearts. "It is good for me to be afflicted so that I might learn your decrees. (Psalm 119)" I put the card on the kitchen counter next to the cheesecake recipe. I get busy afflicting my family. That night at dinner, we eat a Fat Bomb.

I sit with Porter at the table while he eats his high-fat supper and I sip water. Brian has taken Tyler out to eat to have normal food at Applebee's where she will be out of sight of her brother. She returns home carrying her paper menu and two crayons. I have food stashed upstairs and have wolfed down a sandwich I make while Porter is strapped into his high chair.

We eat in shifts so Tyler can have normal food and we eat in our bedrooms so Porter won't see it.

He drinks water constantly. I call the Epilepsy Foundation and the volunteer tells me that the dehydration is the hardest part. "Just have your family member carry a gallon jug around." I picture Porter lugging his jug to day care and sipping water between stints on the jungle gym. I don't have the heart to tell the guy that we're talking about a toddler.

"And watch the hidden dietary derailers!" he says before we hang up. "Drink your whiskey straight!"

By week three we are all ready to drink our whiskey straight. Tyler hides pretzels in her bed and Porter crawls under the table, looking for dropped food. I try to stay grounded, conjuring up Jon Kabat-Zinn's meditation voice about embracing the "unfolding now." In fact, I do well until I find my son wrestling the toothpaste cap off and trying to squirt the Crest in his mouth. Then I find myself screaming, "*No!*"

A few days later he has a seizure. Brian's acknowledgment of the obvious makes me reflexively hostile.

"At least now we can eat at the dining table," he says.

"I think it's the Crest."

"It didn't work. And having a quality of life is as important."

It's hard to argue with that, and I kind of resent him for being so logical. I'm mad he's right, mad we won't be keto-fied, and mad at myself for being mad at my husband again. I'm ruminating about how I'll tell Julie. We agree to try the diet for a few more days. In a few more days, we're in the ambulance headed back to the ER.

I talk to my father late at night. I am down the hall from Porter's hospital room in a lounge with a calling card. It is two hours earlier in California and I catch him after dinner.

"What's happening?" he asks.

I start to cry. "Still in the ICU" is all I can answer.

A minute passes with nothing, just the sound of our breathing.

"I love you," he says.

"I love you," I say back. And then we hang up.

With the renewed episodes, Porter's behavior takes a nosedive and he picks up a new habit. When he is frustrated, he snaps his jaw shut. When I tell him to stop this he bangs his chin on the table, and then cries hysterically. I tell the neurologist that I am worried about his jaw and the doctor says, "Luckily the teeth are the strongest bone in our body."

One day at dinner, Tyler takes charge. I watch her coach him from her seat at the dining table.

"Hitting your head is not the best option when you are frustrated, Porter," she tells him. Porter pauses, then whacks himself again. "When I'm mad, I distract myself." I realize that my five-year-old is providing therapy to her brother. I want to intervene but I'm listening to her, getting pointers.

Porter pauses, mid-hit, his arm still up by his helmet.

"Pay attention, Porter, we are talking about your behavior," she instructs.

"Come in, Christopher Robin!" he says.

"Good job, Porter. That's what I mean. If you want to hit your head, just think about *Winnie the Pooh*." Her advice is logical and I wonder how she's figured this out. I wonder how this child has turned out so well given the conditions she's endured.

Tyler is done with the therapy, but now Porter's engaged. He laughs hysterically and asks, "Where's my daughter?" He asks this a lot. It is guaranteed to make people at the gas station stare.

Tyler plays the straight man. "You don't have a daughter, Porter. I'm sorry to tell you this, but you never will."

16

My father visits me. He is a writer and business consultant and flies around the country to talk about organizational transitions. On his way back from New York, he stays with us and we are both up early in the morning.

My father and I decide to go for a run together after having coffee. We meet in the kitchen. Outside the window, snowflakes ping against the pane. Dad is wearing a T-shirt.

"I think you'll need something warmer, Dad. It's windy out there."

"I'll be okay—I don't get cold very easily."

"How about a sweatshirt—Brian has extra ones?"

"I'll be fine." I shrug my shoulders and bundle up.

We run down 12th Avenue and crisscross the streets into an open area by the lake. The wind whistles and my father abruptly stops. "It's a little painful breathing in this wind!" he says. He has his hand over his chest and doubles over. I mentally run through CPR steps and realize I only know the infant kind.

"It's cold. Here, take one of my sweatshirts." I give my dad a sweatshirt, one of three that I am wearing. He has one and I have two. My father puts it on and we turn around.

"I guess I should have taken you up on the windbreaker," he concedes.

"It's deceptive looking outside."

When we get to the door of my house, Porter is flapping and runs out when we open the door. He runs right past us and into the street. My father chases him and catches him by the arm.

"Hi, Porter," Porter says. Porter keeps running and they both slip and they are hobbling as Dad tries to pull him back. It looks like a three-legged race. Dad kisses his head and Porter flaps. That is like a hug for him.

We stumble inside. "Just say it," he says, laughing.

"What?" I ask.

"Just say it, 'I told you so,'" he insists.

"I'm not going to say that—it was hard to gauge!" I exclaim.

My father goes in the living room and wraps a blanket around him. "You'd think from all those *Little House on the Prairie* books we read, especially *The Long Winter*, that I would have known better."

"It wasn't hyperbole, or it wasn't all hyperbole when she said all those cows froze to death," I tell him.

"Very believable," he responds.

It strikes me that I haven't heard anything more from Porter. Quiet seems nice, but silence usually means he is up to something. I hear a noise behind us and see him sitting on the couch with the remote in his hand. He is holding it backwards and upside-down, pointing it towards the TV and trying to turn on a movie.

Dad smiles. "A triumph of testosterone over brain injury."

Later on, we are warm again after showering and putting on wool socks and slippers. We sit on the floor in the living room, our backs against the couch. We watch Porter as he puts the wooden letters in the puzzle beside him. Apropos of nothing he says, "Dangerous! Don't touch knives." Dad dumps the puzzle and Porter starts over.

"I was rereading *Man's Search for Meaning*. Viktor Frankl can really put things in perspective."

"I can see why you would be reading that now," he responds.

"I think Frankl's idea about finding meaning in what happened to Porter does more for me than anything else," I tell him. "The only problem is that I can't see the meaning. Right now I just see the inside of an ambulance every other week."

"It's hard to know, at this time, what we'll be imprinted from with an experience like this, isn't it?" Dad says.

"All I see at the time, now, is a kid with brain damage, the inside of the ER, and a mother who hasn't made a dent in the whole problem."

"What I see," Dad responds, "is resilience, and coping, and letting go."

We sit like that for another few minutes without talking. We sit like that because there is nothing else to say.

The resilience is less a personality trait than part of my human wiring. There's a whole evolutionary psychology part to this—the crisis-rally-crisis loop. I know that surviving danger is the critical part to actually surviving and every organism is hardwired to do it; even insects have a bug version of dopamine called octopamine that would let them lift cars off of their kids if they had arms. It's why we get through danger and why we think we can survive anything. Even my heroes fell in this trap and I think of Sir Isaac Newton, who killed himself breathing mercury vapors when he tried to turn lead into gold. I'm willing to try things to fix things and nothing is out of bounds. I want to turn lead into gold.

I tell my latest diet plan to my other support group friend, MJ, and she acts as if she gets it. I liked her the minute I met her. Well, not the actual minute I met her, because initially she seemed hostile. It was at the second meeting I attended that I began to like her.

I sat across from her, next to Julie the cheerleader. I was telling Julie how Porter's issues made me feel like an Old Testament character. I eloquently shared a monologue that covered his history, Greek mythology, and a mysterious connection between the two. It may have been a tiny bit hard to follow.

MJ looked at me quizzically, similar to the way in which dogs look at you when you talk to them, and said, "I don't know what the fuck you just said." Five minutes later we were close friends.

MJ is devoutly Christian and swears constantly, which gives her credibility in my book. She grew up in a trailer park and now has returned back to the trailer park since her boyfriend left. Their son was born disabled and he said the relationship wasn't fun anymore.

As we talk on the phone today, I relay all my theories about how we will fix our children. This time I tell her about the Pacific Gyre and big industry and why the Frito-Lay Company is evil.

"Go for it," she says like she always does. "God didn't carry you this far, Sarah, to drop you on your ass."

I go for it.

We overhaul the family's eating habits: The microwave is dumped and processed foods are replaced by a diet my father refers to as "bark and acorns." I am black-and-white: no trans-fats, no food dyes. Brian is always hungry, sneaking Snickers bars from the vending machines in the teachers' lounge at school.

One day when I am out, Tyler asks Amy, the babysitter, "Quick, Mom is gone—can I have some bacon?"

I am a single-minded, sleep-deprived militant, albeit a tired militant. I'm armed with a plan. The new diet stops the seizures.

Porter develops more language skills, but his communication is strange. He says a handful of phrases over and over. One morning, he gets going with, "Hello Mother, hello Mother, hello Mother," in a sweet voice that reminds me of Anthony Perkins in the shower scene in *Psycho.*

When I get Porter ready to leave the house, he holds a foot out to me and says, "Tie your shoe." I'm irritated by the way he becomes locked into phrases, repeating them over and over like a CD skipping.

Porter is also very sweet. Anthony Perkins was probably sweet as a baby, too. I take the children to the park a few days later and see this side. It's the boy that is there beneath all the medications. Porter stands a few feet away, blowing bubbles into a gentle breeze. He walks over to a Golden Retriever lolling in the dust and holds the wand in front of the dog's mouth.

"Blow!" he says. As I watch Porter, it dawns on me that the recipe I've had to right Porter's life had become his life, and perhaps, the brain that needs fixing is mine. The thought comes. The thought goes. Later it comes and it stays.

But the thought isn't sticking yet. It's Saturday morning; by 9:00, Porter has dumped shampoo on the carpet and scribbled on the walls. Then I hear clapping and run into the bathroom to find that he's stuffed the toilet with toothbrushes and Kleenex. He giggles and says, "Don't touch knives," as the bowl overflows.

As I sop up the water with towels, Porter darts past me and throws kibble around the living room, yelling, "*Eat, Dog.*"

We need to get out of the house, so I load the kids into the car to drive to an indoor park while Brian unclogs the toilet. Upon arrival, we pile our coats on a metal bench and line up for the slide.

At the top of the slide steps, a boy Porter's age asks him, "Do you want to go first or should I?" Porter flaps his hands and jumps up and down. Then he turns around and bolts down the steps, knocking over a toddler.

I set her back on her feet and say, "Slow down, Porter." He looks at me and answers, "Hi, Porter."

"Right," I say, "slow down."

Porter climbs on the platform behind him, grabs the fire pole, and jumps. He hangs there, stuck, unable to figure out how to slide to the ground until I lift him down.

"Don't do that," I tell him. A minute later, he is dangling on the pole again. We repeat this four more times until I am distracted taking a drink of water. I look back just in time to see a hearty woman in snow boots falling on her back with Porter on top of her. The only warning she had was when Porter yelled, "Jump!"

"I am sorry," I say, pulling the woman to her feet. She looks dazed. "He's much faster than he looks." I grab our coats and call Tyler to go. She walks over slowly.

"But we just got here," she says.

"I know, but Porter's getting in trouble," I tell her.

"We never stay at the park," she responds, defeated.

"Come on, we need to go."

While unlocking the car I tell Porter to stay by my side, but a moment later he declares, "Home," and heads off across a snowy field. He marches towards a frozen lake. It reminds me of stories I've read of native people who march off in the cold when it is their time. I race to catch up to him, then lead him back to the car and buckle him into the booster seat.

As we make our way out of the parking lot, Tyler asks, "On my birthday can I stay at the park for at least ten minutes?"

Every other week I take Porter to his neurologist to check his medication levels. Because Depakote can cause liver failure, we test him bimonthly to make sure his organs are not on the blink. The offices are part of a hospital and sit in a bad part of town. They are nestled between a payday lender and a pawnshop. There is a church across the street with a menu board with inspiring messages for all the drug addicts in the neighborhood. This week the sign reads WHEN DOING THE IMPOSSIBLE, KEEP YOUR EYES ON HIM, NOT THE CIRCUMSTANCES.

There is a park on the other side but it's empty. I wonder what the park is like when the day is over. I unbuckle Porter and we head for the building. We pass young black men huddled on the corner and they stop talking the minute we're close. I know about unconscious bias, the way white people tense up the minute they see a group of black men. Porter's a white person, but he doesn't tense up; he smiles at them and runs full speed until he's standing in the middle of the group. He jumps in place and holds his hand up to high five the biggest one. He hasn't learned the alphabet, but he learned to high five the first day of preschool. The group stares and Porter holds his hand up again, jumping so the man can see it.

"Sorry," I say, as I run to catch up.

The man ignores me and bends down. He high fives Porter and walks away.

We go along the street behind the office building. The house near the entrance has a living room set on the porch. The couch is sloped and a cushion is missing. There is a sign posted that says they have a dog that bites. I want a sign like that to warm people up, to tell them my son might sip their drink or pull the fire alarm, which he does today in the elevator on the ride up to the doctor.

He yanks the switch and it blares and he laughs, doubled over, as if he'd heard the best joke of his life. Everyone stares. Porter laughs. He tries to grab it again and I intercept his arm. Now he screams. He grabs for it again and I stop him again. The other people give us dirty looks as we ride down to the foyer and again outside while the firemen declare it a drill. I want to explain but I don't, and people look away because Porter is lying on the ground taking off his pants.

"You just need to be firm," a woman says to me. I get this a lot and I've learned to expect it. Her hair is perfect and her child is perfect while my child lies on the ground with his pants around his ankles. We are cleared to go up and as we step on the elevator Porter grabs for the fire alarm. But I am faster. My arms pin his arms and we ride three floors with him kicking his feet and trying to bite me. People stare. He grabs my bra and it snaps and we walk into the waiting room, me with uneven breasts.

I am excited to tell Dr. Garrison about our new cure. He is always receptive and kind. I have a feeling he's worried about me, mentally speaking. We are making the changes as a family and I am all in. In addition to the diet I also switch to natural cleaners and deodorant made of witch hazel. The deodorant is the toughest transition and I keep the real kind, the type with aluminum, in the back of my closet for emergencies.

I explain the plan to him. "Yes, it seems weird, but it works," I say, keeping my arms pinned at my sides. He smiles and I'm not sure if he's being nice or pretending I don't smell, but I go with it and smile back. I feel a bond with our doctor, as we shared the same advisor at the University of Minnesota. He nods with great interest. At the time it seems like we're connecting, but at the time I haven't slept through the night in two years.

The visit ends as it always does, on a bad note. The blood draw happens in a room in the back, where the patient sits in a chair with a tray that folds down like the bar you lock on a carnival ride.

We walk to the room and Porter tenses in my arms. He knows what will happen and he screams before we begin. I sit in the chair and he sits on my lap and we are both strapped in while the technician approaches.

"Don't touch knives!" he screams, because that's what he's heard when he does something dangerous.

"It won't hurt, honey," says the technician. It will hurt and he knows it and he hits her arm when she tries to draw his blood.

I am less consoling and pin his arms to his sides and say, "*Do it, do it!*" like I can hardly wait.

He screams and arches. I squeeze and I hold him and eventually she does it after trying three times. "Geez, what's that for?" Porter asks. Tears streak his face. I get home. I call my mother for moral support and she says it sounds like something is wrong with me. I tell her nothing is wrong which really means everything is wrong. She comes to see us the next week.

She reads to the kids and takes Tyler to lunch. She wants to spend special time with Tyler. I ask her why and she says Tyler needs extra attention.

We pick her up at the airport. My mother kisses the kids, then me. Tyler hisses and claws.

My mother looks concerned. "I hope she isn't feeling like she needs to act out to find a place in the family," she says.

I say, "Uh-huh," or something to that effect. I hope we can drop it.

My mother makes us breakfast the next day. Porter and Brian smile and Tyler doesn't hiss so I feel good. Mom can't help commenting on the natural diet. We eat whole-wheat toast, tofu, and kiwis. Porter loves kiwis.

"Do you think he gets enough protein?" she asks. She has already mentioned that Porter seems short. But she doesn't get that I do not care about protein anymore. Porter has not had a seizure in weeks.

Tyler says, "If Porter's a midget, can you park in the blue parking spaces?"

Porter eats another kiwi.

If he's a seizure-free midget, I can live with that.

My mother begins to make remarks again about going after Big Pharma. I explain that we are in the court system and we can't unless we opt out. Mom thinks it's taking too long. She can't help herself; my mother has the barest tendency towards being provocative and she wants us to step up the pace. She is a worrier even in the best of times and now is worried sick by proxy.

I think my mother is catastrophizing. Then Porter is kicked out of his church day. Then I think that maybe she isn't.

Four years ago they sent him home because he stopped breathing—now he breathes but he won't sit still.

Then kindergarten starts and he isn't ready. I know this because he's tested and doesn't score a single point. Tyler is there. It is Saturday and going for cognitive testing is a family outing.

The evaluation is a combination of facts and problem solving, neither of which is Porter's strong suit. We go to the kindergarten room and sit in tiny chairs, my knees bunched up by my chin. The walls are covered with kids' drawings—the kind with stick bodies and giant bubble heads. There are posters of people smiling with chipper messages. No one wears a helmet.

The woman starts our test with several scenarios. She is earnest. She is young. It's not her fault.

"Okay Porter," she says, "we're going to talk about a few different situations." Porter flaps. Tyler sits at attention.

"I just need you to answer my questions," she says.

"He doesn't answer questions," I say.

"I bet you're underestimating him. Let's give it a try."

I bet I'm not, I think to myself, but we give it a try.

"Okay Porter, what do you do at the end of the day?" *Flap, flap*. Silence.

Teacher scribbles something. Tyler raises her hand.

"Did you want to say something?" the teacher asks.

"You go to bed!" Tyler says and the woman smiles. Tyler has it right since she passed the test just last year, as they are sixteen months apart.

"Let's see if we can get your brother to answer one," she says. Tyler pulls her hand down and puts it around Porter.

"Let's try another one. What happens when you break a friend's toy?"

Silence.

More silence.

Tyler leans over to him and whispers, "Say, 'You go to jail!'"

Porter says, "Jail!" and Tyler claps.

It worries me that Tyler knows about incarceration and I shake my head. Tyler shrugs her shoulders at me and the teacher watches us and jots things down. It worries me that she thinks I've made my children this way.

We switch to the matching game and things look up—Porter knows his name. But he says it at the wrong time.

"What's this?" the woman asks, holding up a picture of a car.

"Hi, Porter," he answers.

She sounds firm. "What's *this*?" she asks again, the way Americans scream louder in English when people from other countries don't speak the language.

He looks at the card and replies, "Hi, Porter."

She pulls another card out of the pile. This one is a flower. "What's this?" she asks him.

"I had pizza for lunch." It's eight in the morning and he didn't have pizza for lunch; in fact, he hasn't had pizza in a year since we changed our diet.

She hasn't quit. She holds up a banana. "How about this one?"

"I had pizza for lunch," he responds.

Tyler takes charge. "That's a banana, Porter. Say 'banana.'"

"Nana," says Porter.

"Very good, Porter. Yes, that's a banana!" Tyler claps. Porter claps. The woman puts down the pile of cards.

"Alrighty!" she says, and I see her write a zero next to the last question. There is a column of zeroes above it. It seems like she should shield the scores or use a euphemism so the absence is less obvious.

"I don't think he's on track for kindergarten," she says.

"Probably not," I say. I want her to know I get it, that I'm not one of those parents that claims their disabled kid is normal and should be taking calculus with everyone else. I force a smile.

"We will look at options and get back to you," she says and stacks up her papers. I stand up. Tyler grabs her brother's hand.

"Sorry Porter, you got an 'F,' but don't feel bad. I'll teach you the flash cards at home."

17

FOUR YEARS

We go for a checkup with Dr. Cohen. Ostensibly this is aimed at tracking progress. In the absence of progress we leave with a new diagnosis: Porter has autism.

"This may be difficult to hear," he says as we sit in plastic chairs next to his desk. There are blocks and books and a tray of plastic animals. "It is apparent that Porter has severe delays."

"Got it." I sound impatient. I know that, but it doesn't help.

"Keep going," I say. I know what he is going to tell me.

"You've brought up autism and that is clearly the diagnosis."

I look at Porter in the corner of the room pouring beads from cup to cup.

"I've evaluated his speech, behavioral patterns, social interactions, and cognitive testing," he continues, "and everything signals this diagnosis." I think of Porter's echolalia, hand flapping, jaw clamping, and tantrums. The label is not a surprise.

But the label also scares me. My earliest association with it stems from my childhood.

When my mother studied to be a therapist she did her training at a psychiatric facility. Mom described one unusual patient who would spend the day banging his head against the metal window frame. Once he hit it so hard he had to have his skull stitched up. She told us about it one night after work, the blood stains from his gash still visible on her shirt. He had a condition she'd never seen before. He had autism.

I squirm in my chair as the words sink in. My feelings are nowhere to be found.

Feel something, I think.

Zip.

I am not sure if I should be happy to know what's wrong or sad to have the facts. Next to me Porter flaps his hands as he finishes a puzzle.

Dr. Cohen and I are done and he squeezes my shoulder as I leave. I hold Porter's hand as we walk through the corridors. A man in a wheelchair rolls past us and we go through the heavy doors to the parking lot. We walk in silence until we get to the car. As I lift him into his car seat he smiles at me.

"Busy day!" he says.

"Busy day," I say back.

Dr. Cohen says that he will send a report to our doctors and write another in support of our vaccine claim. I call Katherine the minute we are home.

"Dr. Cohen says he has autism," I tell her.

"Wow. That has to be hard to hear," she responds. She's sympathetic but not surprised.

"It is and it isn't. It's relieving to have a name for what is happening."

"We'll include it with the case materials. Will he write up a report?"

"He will have it to you by the end of the week."

We wrap up our discussion and I wait for Brian to get home. I tell him about the new diagnosis before he walks through the door and has a chance to set his things down.

"Maybe we can finally get him services," he says.

"It's weird to have that kind of label. Does that worry you?" I feel my post-traumatic stress welling up. *My son has autism*, I think.

"He's still Porter. The label will just help us figure out resources." I nod my head. I am uncharacteristically quiet.

"He's still the same person," he says again.

18

It's strange that my husband and I love each other, but can't stand to be in the same room. I don't know if we fight because we have marriage problems or have marriage problems because we fight. Maybe Porter can't be normal, but our family can, and I want Tyler to have a regular childhood and a regular sibling, the kind who will respond to her questions with real answers, not just *Winnie the Pooh* quotes.

It's the absence of touching that I noticed first. Brian and I go through the motions of family time, like actors playing the part of a married couple. We sleep on opposite sides of the bed, and getting along has been redefined as a night without arguing. Some nights we fight about fighting.

"You don't understand," I say. "Our constant fighting is a bad sign." I am mad again. Also I'm exhausted and this is Brian's fault.

"You don't understand," he replies. "We don't constantly fight."

I focus on all of the things Brian is doing wrong. Focusing on Brian is my first thought, because I can't get mad at my son. The voice in my head is a running commentary, blabbing nonstop like the CNN weather report. The blabbing makes it hard to notice how I'm coming across and doesn't help stop thoughts like, *throw Brian under the bus when you're mad.*

My thoughts are self-referential and oblivious, and it isn't the first time I've missed my impact. In class a few months back we had a mock group therapy session and within five minutes the professor singled me out. I don't even use profanity regularly, but something about the therapy setting gave me the urge to swear. It was as if I had Tourette's and found myself saying something offensive every four minutes.

My behavior was pointed out, but I didn't get it. The professor was so subtle and Minnesotan that I didn't realize she was talking to me. In fact, I was thinking, *Geez, people really should be more considerate,* until I realized everyone was staring at me. I flipped in that moment from feeling good and maybe the tiniest bit superior, to feeling a little like I'd wandered into class without my pants on.

This crosses my mind as I fight with Brian about who started the fight. I stop and we stop. We make up.

We decide that the problem between us is the relentless pressure and that a vacation might bang things back into shape. We decide we are going to make this work and we head off for a weekend to talk about the future. Brian's parents come babysit and we fly to Las Vegas where it's warm and far away.

The long weekend is luxurious. We sleep nine hours each night and walk along the strip holding hands. In the mornings we jog as the city awakens, weaving around a tourist staggering home drunk. We stop at 24-hour buffets and drink ninety-nine cent coffee out of cups emblazoned with the Hoover Dam. I look at my husband as we read the paper, trading sections without talking. I realize how much we enjoy each other. I realize why we are married.

We talk about what is happening. Apparently a full night's sleep lets you do it without arguing. I forgot that Brian is funny.

Now I am sitting next to him laughing. *We are going to make this work,* I think. We recommit to the future and to each other.

We also decide that we will have one more baby.

Everyone thinks we've lost it and this is a crazy idea. I know that for a fact when I tell MJ the news and she says, and I quote, "Have you lost it?" Part of the problem is that I have trouble articulating why this is a good time to get pregnant. There is a grain of logic in the question and I make a mental list of the pros and cons.

Pro: I want Tyler to have a sibling she can talk to.
Con: We are at the hospital every few weeks.
Con: Nobody sleeps through the night.
Pro: We will already be up when the baby awakens.
Con: We are constantly stressed.
Con: The new baby's brother was kicked out of day care before he was two.
Con: The new baby's sister thinks you go to jail when you break a toy.

The pros win out, since the cons aren't ever considered. Secretly, there is more to it than that. I want a chance to make up for what happened to Porter. It doesn't matter how many times I've been told that bad things just happen and nothing I did directly caused this. In my head, I tell myself, *my child has problems = I am a bad mother.*

No matter how much I understand intellectually that this isn't the case, a part of me still faces the firing squad. Without the ability to reverse the clock, I look for a way to do the experience over. I want to fix what happened by having a healthy child and by doing everything right this time around. If the denominator (number of healthy children) gets bigger, then my bad-mother score has to get smaller. It has to make things better for all of us.

And just like that, we conceive. In roughly five minutes. I stop taking the birth control pills and two weeks later, I am pregnant. I am determined to do everything right for the next baby. *I will balance the scales for the family,* I tell myself. It starts with my pregnancy diet—when Brian stops at the grocery store on the way home, I give him my list: "Spinach, lean meat, fruits, and cheese. *No junk food!*"

Brian glances at it and asks, "What's this?"

"I'm off sugar. And can you get those eggs from the chickens that listen to classical music?"

MJ doesn't let up about how much of a bad idea a new baby is and quotes the comic Jim Gaffigan, "Having a third kid is like drowning and someone hands you a baby." She says it firmly, but she means it nicely. It doesn't affect me. I want to redress what happened. I want to save my marriage. I am convinced that another baby will bond our family back together. We will land on our feet.

Katherine calls a few days later to say, "The government wants you to rerun Porter's metabolic screen and EEG. They think it is inconclusive."

"We just did the EEG a month ago," I say, realizing I am arguing with my ally. "Isn't it still good?"

"Apparently something raised a flag for the government doctor." I'm learning firsthand about the problem of too many tests. False positives are never positive, but with enough procedures they occur a lot.

We rerun all the tests and the results are clear, meaning no findings. The government wants to find something that points the blame away from the vaccine. We measure and test and things do turn up, but then become dead-ends. None of the paths lead to anywhere real.

A day after that, I am back to my research. I am in a nursing home to observe patients with dementia and physically aggressive behavior. I sit in one of the folding chairs by the piano and observe the interaction at the nurses' station. I see a woman that I have tested many times, named Melinda, and realize she has transitioned to the locked Alzheimer's ward.

Melinda is across the hall talking to another patient, telling her about the dangers of carnival rides. "A man was riding the Ferris wheel and a Canada goose flew right into his head. It was flapping, you know, migrating somewhere, and it almost tore his neck off."

I can hear the nurse muttering something, but Melinda interrupts. "So everyone is going on and on about the man's neck injury and the dangers of those rides, but no one mentions the goose. Not one person mentioned the bird. So my question is, 'What about the goose?' It probably had a neck injury too. Why wouldn't they give any kind of update on its health? Do you think the paper could release that kind of information if I called?"

The other woman shakes her head and Melinda says, "You're forgetting about the Freedom of Information Act." She is still for a minute, then looks at a man strapped into his wheelchair.

She shakes him to wake him up. "Do you think this is a cover-up? Are they hiding information about the bird?" she asks him.

I am thinking of myself. This never ends well. It reminds me of Poe's story of William Wilson and the split between man's self and observer. I proceed through my day and watch from the sidelines, making helpful mental comments like—*nothing is getting better.*

Later that night I cuddle with Tyler when we get home from the library and open *Alice in Wonderland.* I read aloud, "You used to be much more . . . 'muchier.' You've lost your muchness."

"What is your muchness?" she asks. If she were a reporter, she'd be jotting it in her notebook and I watch her watch me. My observer is in charge and I try to think of a good answer.

"The stuff inside," I say.

Observer says, *weak answer.*

"Like God?" she asks.

Observer says, *a deep answer is needed.*

"Yes, the most important part of us."

Observer says, *lame.*

Tyler is quiet. "Is that what you think?" I ask.

"Yes, like Porter," she says. "He is very muchy. Sometimes his muchness just bursts out and makes him flap."

Observer says, *more insightful than your answers.*

"You're right, sometimes it does," I say, because usually I don't know how to respond to her questions. And because I have lost my muchness and wish I was muchier.

Tyler and I read one chapter and then another. It is peaceful because Porter is in the corner with his LEGO table, stacking the blocks into intricate towers. I love the LEGOs and I hate the LEGOs. I love the LEGOs because he loves the LEGOs and I hate them because he is very territorial. For a few weeks I brought him to the health club with me on Saturdays; he and Tyler would play in the childcare center while I went for a run. This was a great solution since it was seven degrees below zero outside. And then it was a bad solution because Porter couldn't share the LEGOs and then hit another boy who tried to play with them.

This all ended when a rattling voice called my name. I heard the loud speaker as I jogged along. "Sarah Bridges, please come to the child center." This could be bad or this could be awful, and I jumped off the treadmill and went down.

I see Porter in the corner and he is throwing something—they're LEGOs. The teacher is standing a few feet away with her arms crossed.

"He won't share with the other children," she says.

"You go that way!" Porter responds.

She continues. "I explained he has to take turns and he threw a LEGO at me. He hit me in the eye."

"You said that!" Porter replies. He turns his back and hunches over his tower.

"I'm sorry," I say.

"We can't have violent children in the center," she tells me.

"He doesn't understand that they aren't his alone," I say. If this were a Poe story, he would write one part showing me apologizing and then another part where I could say how ineffective that was. If this were a Poe story, we'd have a beginning, middle, and end, and the story would most likely lead to murder. I think this is a Poe story.

The teacher isn't done. "You should teach him to share."

Now Tyler has joined the scene and she has her arms crossed too. I have that effect on people.

"Autistic kids like to play alone," Tyler explains. She is a four-foot-six social worker and the teacher is stumped. Tyler has this effect on people.

"I warned him before I took the LEGOs away and he ignored me." She is mad he won't listen. "He threw them at me. He'll take out an eye."

I scoop up Porter. His arms swing and his legs kick and the teacher follows us out of the room.

"He can't come back," she says.

"He can't come back," Tyler says. Porter kicks, the teacher stares, and we walk out. We don't go back.

Now I am sitting across from our pediatrician, Dr. Amit, the same one that came to the hospital years ago when Porter was brain damaged. We're in for our well-child appointment and it's time for booster shots.

I beat her to the punch. "Vaccines are safe," I say. This startles her and she looks up.

"Yes, they are perfectly safe, however the CDC has new guidelines and we don't give the pertussis vaccine to children who had a bad outcome," she says.

I look at Porter; he's in his helmet, lying under my chair with his shirt pulled up. He's scribbled circles on his chest with a pen.

"I'm guessing we qualify," I say.

I am thinking about the CDC guidelines. I am familiar with them, as I check the website each week. In fact, just this morning I read the CDC release about a new study that was published. "Concerns about the safety of whole-cell pertussis vaccines prompted development of acellular vaccines that are less likely to provoke adverse events because they contain purified antigenic components of Bordetella pertussis."[16] It's in a study that says the acellular version is ready for prime time and they're rolling it out for babies.

I am six months pregnant and eating organic spinach and avoiding preservatives, and playing classical music as I type up papers for my graduate classes. Things seem to be going well with *this* child, but I am worried about our unborn baby. He doesn't move for a day and I call the OBGYN. The doctor knows what we've gone through with Porter and tells me to come in for an ultrasound. I could easily be overthinking it. I know this intellectually, but it makes no difference. I head to the doctor's office for a visit.

I lie on the table and yank up my shirt. My physician rubs gel on my belly and puts the sonar against my skin. Images leap onto the screen and the doctor stands beside me, studying the pictures. I wait for the bad news.

"Well, I see a baby boy lying on his back sucking his thumb," he tells me.

"Is he alive?" I ask.

"Very much so. He looks quite relaxed, like he's in a hammock on the beach."

---

16 CDC. Pertussis Vaccination: Use of Acellular Pertussis Vaccines Among Infants and Young Children Recommendations of the Advisory Committee on Immunization Practices (ACIP). MMWR March 28, 1997.

"Then why hasn't he moved in the past day? That seems like a bad sign." I'm still worried.

"I'll tell you my opinion based on anecdotal experience. Often the laid-back babies turn into laid-back people. I think maybe you just have a go-with-the-flow personality on the way," he explains.

I am relieved to hear this. The doctor studies the screen a bit longer. I imagine he is trying to remember his genetics classes and decipher how it is that a neurotic mother gives birth to a Zen practitioner. I get off the table and stop worrying about the baby. By that I mean I don't make any more anxious phone calls to the doctor for the rest of the pregnancy.

19

5 YEARS

There is a special school that I learn about from the speech therapist Porter sees on Tuesdays. It is a place where half the kids are like Porter. It is a school for distracted letter-hating children with seizures. We hurry to get Porter on the waiting list and meet with the woman who runs the program.

"What a sweetie," she says when Porter hugs her leg. He likes to do that, to hug strangers' legs. People usually jump when he does it but she doesn't. "The intake process involves an assessment of Porter and an interview with our psychologist. She's terrific."

"What kind of assessment?" I ask.

"Just a basic developmental test to see which classroom is the best place for him." I wait for her to grab the flash cards, but instead she asks, "What does he like to do for fun?"

"LEGOs. Building towers."

"He'll fit right in."

On the first day, he does fit right in, just like she said. A month later there is a ceremony with the students and parents. The children sit in a circle on the ground in the gym. We parents are in the bleachers clapping like it's the Academy Awards. I see Porter on the floor next to a girl in a wheelchair. The teachers are giving out medals and there is a prize for everyone. They walk or wheel themselves to the middle of the room to have them placed around their necks. Porter wins for basketball since he makes his shot almost every time. When they call his name he stares across the room blankly. A teacher in running shoes grabs his hand and brings him up to the podium.

"Good job, Porter!" the teachers say. He leans over to the microphone like the other kids. Everyone else said thank you.

The principal hugs him and I can't help it—I yell, "Way to go Porter!" He hears my voice and looks towards me. He leans closer to the microphone. His breathing echoes over the loudspeaker like an obscene phone call. He looks me in the eye.

"Don't pick your nose, Mommy," he says. Then he walks back to his seat.

Our focus on doing everything right this time continues after our baby, Jackson, arrives: We carry him everywhere, he sleeps in our bed, and I nurse him for a full year. He has a relaxed personality. The day he turns three months old, I watch him as he lies across my lap, smiling, and it strikes me—getting it right for Jackson has brought something good and light to the family.

I watch him smile and suck his thumb, and as long as he's healthy I don't mind if he does that for the next twenty years. I still need to check when he's asleep that he's doing important things like breathing. I lounge around the house for his first three months barely cracking the front door. Putting on my bathrobe is considered getting dressed. I am euphoric that he is here and ecstatic that he is healthy and we spend hours of each day grinning at each other on the couch.

It is a week before our trial begins. I wonder how we will take Porter on a plane. Then Katherine calls me, "You've won your case." I am sitting in our living room watching Porter stack

LEGOs. "The government has agreed that the vaccine caused Porter's brain injury. We are not going to trial."

We are done. I get off the phone and dial Brian. Then my father. We've won the case! I look at Porter in the corner in his helmet and diaper he still wears around the clock. Surprisingly, I don't feel like a winner. There has to be more. I keep rereading the letter in fear that I've missed something. I know the large amount of people waiting for their cases to be acknowledged by the government, people who haven't crossed the finish line. I find it impossible to believe that this letter is stating that we are done. It's impossible.

I think of the mustard gas experiments I learned about in graduate school. The "man break" experiments entailed 2,500 Navy men being locked in a room and doused in mustard gas to test the effects on the human body. The soldiers were African American, as they wanted to see if dark skin held greater immunity, or less power. Whatever the case, the effects, predictably, were bad.

The worst part is that there was never any acknowledgment of the damage and torture put upon these men. For five decades the Pentagon kept the experiments classified and threatened the men to never disclose what had happened. When the truth finally surfaced, the battle began. The injured veterans, muddling along with disabilities, had to prove their ailments resulted from the poisonous exposure. The government created a table with mustard gas–related health problems, but forced the men to rule out other causes. As they tried to prove it, they were told they'd be prosecuted under the Espionage Act if they went public. They tried to prove their illnesses were poison-induced, but the government fought back that they failed to meet the criteria.

Only after severe pressure from the veterans did the government say they would pay for their health bills. Unfortunately, the payments never came and the men began to die as they grew older and sicker.

In our case, the table for vaccine injuries exists. In our case, Porter's injuries will be compensated. But just like the soldiers in the man break trials, no one ever speaks out to acknowledge the harm. We are told to sign the settlement papers.

Even though we've won our case, we are not done. Phase two entails a process of documentation and expert testimony aimed to detail the specifics of Porter's future needs. This piece requires answering the question, *How much does it cost to raise a child with autism, mental retardation, intractable seizures, and behavioral problems?*

Enter the life care planner. I like that the word "care" is part of the title and picture a nurturing grandmother tallying his needs. Then she visits us. Exit grandma and bring in the actuary, as the process is more about statistics than an examination of Porter's life. I reassure myself that the HHS is on our side now that causality is settled. Vaccines have side effects and so we have the vaccine court. Damaged children have special needs and so we have life planners.

The future need predictions must be exhaustive because the money available is allotted now and can't be amended in the future. As a result, we scrutinize the waterfront: drugs, hospitalizations, ambulance rides, diapers, wheelchairs, helmets, and group homes.

There are two ways to approach the phase: We can hire a planner and the government will, too, or we can share one that HHS provides. The government pushes for sharing the person they designate as a single point of contact, and in fact this is advised in guidelines that accompany the vaccine act. "This results in faster resolution of damages," it reads. It makes sense. One person calling the shots has got to be faster than two.

It makes sense in a collaborative process but doesn't make sense when it is more like a bad divorce. It appears that our case has not unfolded the way those passing the original act envisioned.

The VICP kicked into gear in 1987 and after a year in operation, there were 201 claims. One hundred and sixty-five of these were for the DPT vaccine. The rapid and non-adversarial justice promised by the original law worked well in the early days. The idea was to be non-litigious and that the HHS would be the respondent. One requirement of the act was that HHS would promulgate the program to get the word out to the public of its existence. Once a case was filed, a neutral physician would review the documentation and rule for or against a verdict of vaccine injury.

In the act's first year, the letter of the law was followed and cases were won by default. The act specifies that decisions are reached within 240 days or the case is decided in favor of the petitioner. HHS stated that they failed to have the resources to process the cases and requested that the Department of Justice (DOJ) lawyers defend the cases. With the entry of governmental lawyers, the cases took a turn. In addition to building a defense for the vaccine claim, the neutral arbitrating physician was replaced by trained experts hired to argue against a vaccine-injury diagnosis. In other words, the government hired experts to discredit the injuries that parents brought forth.

Given the challenges we've faced, Katherine recommends getting our own planner. "The last case I settled, the government argued with us over the number of diapers an incontinent teenager needed. I think we want our own expert." The process is dicey, as it requires that we extrapolate out from a five-year-old to determine everything from future medical bills to education or employment status.

We dig in to another government administrative process, which Katherine describes as "being stuck in rush hour traffic for a few months." She doesn't do a great job of selling it.

Before the government's life care planner for HHS visits, the woman wants documentation to determine Porter's needs.

This sounds familiar. It is the usual suspects plus a set of new criteria. Katherine sends us the list: all medical records, doctor visits, lab tests, genetic tests, pregnancy records, well-baby visits, telephone logs, 9-1-1 calls, emergency records, vaccination history, ambulance bills, physical therapy notes, occupational therapy notes, school records, day care reports, pharmacy files, over-the-counter expenditures, monitor fees, insurance records, out-of-pocket expenses, uncovered bills, affidavits from doctors, and "other data as needed."

Then we hit a road bump. The receipts we send need to be validated against file information. Our case is so old that most of the files have been expunged. Our only solution is to contact the organizations one by one and pay to have them examine the information in their microfiche files.

I start with the ambulance company and send in an intern named April to help out. "You really should have saved your receipts," she says.

"We did save them," I tell her. "We just need them corroborated with the company file."

"Bummer." It's never good when a sentence ends that way. "Big bummer," she adds. Even worse. "We don't have things going back that far. I guess our company should have kept our receipts!" April holds her hand over the receiver and says something muffled, then comes back and says, "But I can pull some strings." I have no idea what this means and don't ask and a few weeks later the receipts arrive in the mail.

The materials we've collected so far may not be enough, as the act reads, "In general, any question about relevancy of medical records and the need for production are resolved in favor of production." In other words, *get used to the rush hour traffic.* The government has the right to ask for anything that "might shed light" on our claim. A notation says this is to keep things expeditious and very flexible.

The rationale for setting it up is that it is faster to acquiesce to any request than get bogged down by making the special master referee blow by blow.

We turn in the records. Our file is incomplete. We get more records. Still incomplete. Get more. More to get.

Tyler starts first grade. Our not-so-new baby Jackson is one. He began walking at 9 months and begins to say words. Each day Jackson has more speech and Porter has less. When we go to the open house at our day care they say that Jackson has a number of new tricks.

"Just yesterday he was lying on his back in the gym and throwing a tennis ball in the air and catching it with the same hand!" Brianna likes us again because Jackson is easy and Porter is gone.

I see Brian in the morning before work and then we meet up at the end of the day. We keep notes on Porter's medicines and seizures and appointments. We have spells of constant togetherness when we all spend the day in the emergency room when Porter is hurried in after a seizure. We are effective business partners except when we fight. We fight because it is easier to be mad than to be sad. I can't tell exactly when the marriage broke apart. I can only say that it was wrong side up. The best parts were squashed to the ground. But the medical problems, hospital visits, the tension and worry would not take a holiday. Life without a break does bad things to a family. The pieces and possibilities for a better life folded up and left. Our intimacy is deferred. There isn't a taste of it left in my mouth. Then the intimacy is gone. The marriage is sucked away from me with the same swiftness that wracked Porter's brain. Just like that, it vanishes.

We divorce because it is easier to be sad and alone than to see it reflected every day in the other person.

We finally stop fighting when Brian moves out. It's like the joke about fixing a sore finger by hitting yourself in the head with a hammer. The mechanics of the move go smoothly, but the internal process is raw and jagged. He packs his car and drives away and I wonder how we've constructed this life that we can barely tolerate.

20

The month after Brian moves out, the family is back together in our living room to meet the life care planner. Brian and I sit across from each other on the floor next to the kids.

Tyler reads a book, Jackson plays his xylophone and sings, and Porter pours dried kidney beans from one bowl to another. We don't talk. We are in the midst of writing our divorce decree and starting to write Porter's life care plan.

We are quiet. Nobody hates anyone else. We are bonded together and that is why it is hard to explain to Tyler why we need to be apart.

For the tenth time, I begin to explain that we are getting a divorce. Tyler stops the proceedings. "But, when will Dad move back in?"

"He won't," I start to answer. Tyler cuts in before I surface for air.

"But after that, when will you come back, Daddy?"

"We are living in two houses now. I know this is really hard and we both love you forever," I tell her. "That doesn't change."

Tyler goes back to her book. "Forever isn't always forever."

I say nothing.

A few minutes later we hear a car in the driveway.

The government life care planner is named Shelly and she spends thirty minutes with Porter. In this half hour she will determine all of his financial needs for the next fifty-four years. I don't come up with that number myself. It's from the actuarial table the government uses. There is a formula with bonus points and things that subtract years from Porter's life expectancy. Disease free: plus column. Daily seizures: minus. Injuries from seizures: minus. Not breathing during long seizures: minus. Heart attack during seizures: minus. I never see the formula that leads to the magic number: death.

Shelly says that we should try diet modifications. "Some of the people I've met have worked wonders—" she tells us.

"Are you a vegetarian or carnivore?" Tyler asks. Shelly looks stumped, by the question or maybe by the questioner.

We continue by itemizing needs. We don't fight over future hospitalizations, but we do argue over ambulance rides. As MJ says, "Get a fast car for those trips."

Shelly agrees with us that he is disabled, but we don't agree about his future career. Porter wears a helmet and is unconscious often several times a day, so I am surprised to see that she predicts a job.

"Not a highly professional one," she says. I try to picture a non-professional one, and imagine Porter driving backhoes or bagging groceries. Or maybe a hospital job since he's there so often.

"What kind of job are you seeing?" I ask.

Shelly smiles and closes her folder. "You'd be surprised at the employment people have even when disabled. I imagine you are underestimating his potential."

I look at Porter who is banging his chin on the edge of the coffee table.

It goes along the same path on each need: we agree he has echolalia, but speech therapy is out. A chart has surfaced in which he scrapes the bottom of normal and there's the theoretical possibility that he will still be like a normal kid.

When we get to the part of the questionnaire that addresses communication, she says, "I don't see speech therapy because he is still in the normal range."

"That's funny. That's funny, that's funny," Porter says.

"That's funny," I say. "I don't see a lot of normal day-to-day."

Shelly smiles. "Sometimes things look worse than they actually are. Kids outgrow a lot of things." He's five years old, in diapers, and the neurologist says this is likely a permanent condition. Shelly has a different view, and feels confident he'll be toilet trained in a year.

"What about his seizures?" I ask. "He wets his pants every time he has one." She doesn't answer. She doesn't answer, but we haven't agreed. I've finally caught on that Minnesotans say no by saying nothing and that silence is code for disagreement. I know we haven't agreed when she says the diaper allowance ends in twelve months. I'm fairly certain this proves my point.

Shelly is done with Porter and we are done with Shelly. She packs up her satchel, gets down on a knee to Porter's height, and holds out her hand. Porter picks up his bean bowl and hits her in the face.

Shelly stands back up.

"Alrighty then. We'll work on the plan and have a draft to you next week."

Brian and I continue to live in different houses and trade the kids back and forth on Sundays. It was during one of my weeks with the kids that Porter is hit by a car. I take them grocery shopping and buckle Porter into his seat. As I turn to load groceries he wriggles out, slips through my arms, and dashes into the street. I call his name, and it seems to hang in the air, and in the next moment I hear brakes squeal and Porter scream. An old man's voice yells, "Oh my God!"

I drop the groceries and run around to the car, asking the man, "Was he hit?" Porter is crumpled on the street. Cars stop and people gather around us as I kneel on the wet pavement, holding him in my arms.

A woman bends down and says in my ear, "An ambulance is on its way, hang in there."

"Mama," Porter whimpers. I take off his helmet and lie on the ground holding him. People pull blankets out of their cars and I am struck by how practical Midwesterners are. Porter clutches his foot and cries.

The police arrive first, then the ambulance. An officer stands over us and jots down information in a tiny notebook he pulls from his breast pocket.

He asks, "Are you alright until the EMT gets here?"

Porter is screaming and I am not sure if it is from pain or the fact that I won't let him free.

"We can make it until they come," I respond.

"How did it happen?"

"He's autistic and hyperactive."

He closes his pad. "It was an accident, then."

We are back in the ambulance again, but for a different reason. I sit on the bench to the side of the stretcher and Porter reaches and screams. He grabs his foot and cries. The EMT says to hold him still and I try. He stretches and grabs, and I think how much easier the rides are when he seizes. This is wrong to think and I stop myself. A foot will heal. The seizures don't heal. Porter screams and he reaches and I want to tell him no but I stop myself.

Brian meets me in the ER and takes Jackson onto his lap. Tyler is sitting at the triage desk talking with a nurse. I get closer and hear her say, "How have you been?" and I realize they know each other and are catching up like friends.

Brian and I assume our roles and we don't talk because we are getting divorced. We know our parts and we play them. It's a silent movie and we've seen this part before, but we play our roles anyway.

There is a curtain hanging in the middle of the room to separate our family from the other patient. He is an old man and is confused and asks for his mother. Tyler peers under the curtain, lying on her back.

"Mother? Mother? Where are you, Mother?" he cries, and then he stops midsentence and says, "Who are you down there?" Tyler is caught and she scoots under the curtain on the floor as if she's doing the backstroke on the cement.

"I'm Tyler and my brother was run over by a car because he's autistic and doesn't listen to my mother and runs into traffic and now he has a cast. How are you?"

The old man is quiet. Then he says, "I'm fine. I think. What do you think?"

A doctor comes in and holds a hand out to Porter and Porter ignores him and grabs the glasses off his face. I apologize and hand them back and he does an initial examination indicating that Porter's foot is broken, but he is otherwise all right.

"Good thing he wasn't hit in the head and we aren't dealing with a brain injury," the doctor says. Tyler perks up at this.

"He already has one." Then she leans closer to him and whispers, "That's why he wears the helmet." The doctor seems surprised. He's confused, but I've lost my enthusiasm for telling the story.

Porter gets a walking cast and a pep talk about laying low. We hobble out to the car and get home at 10:00 p.m. Jackson is asleep in his baby seat in the living room and Tyler is brushing her teeth.

I carry Porter into his bed and he tugs on the top of his cast.

"Stuck!" he says.

After putting the other kids to bed I go back to Porter's room and lie down beside him. We sleep like that, in his twin bed, cuddled up in a ball.

21

7 YEARS

Porter is seven years old; the court case is six. We've won our vaccine case, but still haven't worked out the details of the financial settlement. I live in the same house and Brian lives two blocks away. We are divorced, apart, yet see each other every day. Our children go back and forth, one week on and one week off, like commuters.

Everything changes after Porter is hit by the car. The thought enters my mind and stays: *We can no longer take care of Porter alone.* The morning I first considered it I called in sick to work because Porter had been up much of the night, prowling the house. By breakfast he had a seizure, which makes it impossible for him to go to his special education class. By lunchtime, Porter was bored of the sand at the park and climbed the jungle gym. A minute later he had a seizure, falling off the platform and landing in the sand below. I run to him and hold him on my lap until the shaking stops. I attempt to pick him up, but as a large seven-year-old he is more difficult to carry. We sit under the slide for forty-five minutes, waiting for him to wake up.

I look at my watch and realize I am late to get Tyler and have no way to reach the school and tell them what happened. Jackson whines beside me and pulls on my shirt to be held. I decide we have to go, hoist Porter over a shoulder, and balance Jackson on a hip. With stops and starts we make it to the car, only to realize I'd left my purse with the key in it back at the park.

I flag a woman over and ask if she will go to the playground and find my bag. She stares at us for a moment—Porter in his diaper passed out on my lap, Jackson on the ground with a blanket over his face, and then nods and runs back to the park. Then I sit on the curb and watch the other families walk to the park in their flip-flops.

A mother turns to her son and says, "Keep up, honey, you always walk so slowly." The boy skips along, kicking a beach ball ahead of him. I strain to watch them until they disappear over the hill; I can still hear him laughing even after he is gone.

Through MA-TEFRA we are connected to a Minneapolis social worker who is responsible for ensuring that Porter receives the right city services. Porter already has a hospital and school social worker and now has one through the city. I wonder if they ever talk to each other.

Our social worker, Lillian, comes over one day to visit and assess our utilization of services through the city. I imagine they want to know how one child can need so much. It strikes me that they have us on a watch list as cheats that are milking the system. The social worker sent me a checklist before our discussion and I hold it in my lap with my comments and marks. Lillian comes in and we sit on the floor next to Porter and discuss the list.

"It looks like you've marked autism, seizures, behavior problems, school issues, getting along with friends, hygiene, anger management, daily skills, coping, speech problems, and mental retardation," she says, reading from the list.

"Yes," I say, looking at the list in her lap. "The only one I left off was substance abuse. We still have time."

"And he was hit by a car last month?"

I grimace. It is obvious I don't have my act together.

She answers for me. "That must have been traumatic."

"It almost seemed inevitable. Last year I had a man knock on our door and say, *Do you know there is a small child on your roof?* It was wintertime and Porter snuck out the sliding door, climbed up on the woodpile, and onto the low part of the garage. Apparently he wanted to check out the chimney."

She nods. "This is really hard." The non-judgmental look on her face does more for me than any service she might bring.

"How do you relate to the other social workers Porter has?" I ask.

"It is confusing," she says. "There are more than eighty county units in Minnesota and we all operate a little differently. Sometimes we collaborate as a team—that tends to work well. Sometimes I operate on my own and then report back to the disability worker. Usually it boils down to money."

"We have a settlement through the vaccine court," I start. "We have a settlement coming and it will pay for all of the services, in theory, once the fund pays out." The latest thing we've heard from the government is that an annuity is being established and will begin paying for Porter's care in a month. It is a use-it-or-lose-it system, where the account is filled each year and any leftovers go back to the fund. I have a feeling we will use it.

"Then we have some options," she tells me.

I have always liked options, but I have lost my faith in having faith. I nod.

"Let me do some work on this. If anyone qualifies for serious support, Porter does. I will do everything I can."

I like her. I believe her. I have no idea what I hope will happen.

Two weeks later, I invite Lillian over for dinner to ask her advice. Her advice is that Porter needs around-the-clock care, but that the state doesn't support out-of-home placements.

"Then we'll figure it out at home," I say.

She doesn't think the state will back us on any other option. And she doesn't think Porter can manage at home.

Six weeks later, after an evening with the family, Lillian says, "There is a woman in town that specializes in taking care of autistic children. She's done amazing things with some of the kids and is the best there is. Let me speak with her."

What I don't know at the time is that this woman, Ramona, recently decided to stop taking new children. Each placement represents a potential ten- to fifteen-year commitment, and she thought it might be a good time to take a break from such care. But our social worker persists, and Ramona agrees to meet us.

Months later, when I ask Ramona what changed her mind about taking on a new child, she says simply, "I met Porter." On the day of our first visit, Ramona greets me at the door of her three-story Victorian house, barefoot and with a warm smile, holding back the two dogs yapping behind her. She invites me in and sits down to talk, not stopping until the sunlight fades outside.

I visit Ramona again a week later and spend an afternoon with her. As we talk, she tells me about another child she cared for.

"He was five when he moved in here and never spoke," she said. "The doctors thought he wasn't able to because of abuse he'd suffered. We worked at it for quite a while and I was able to get him to open up." Ramona leans forward. "What the doctors don't know is how he first started talking."

"How?" I ask.

"I was driving with him and heard a siren behind us, which I pointed to and said, 'Oh look, there's a police car.' He smiled sweetly and turned to look. As the squad car passed us, he stuck his head out the window and yelled, 'Motherf***ing pigs!' That was my clue that he could talk if he wanted to."

As we speak, Jacob, who lives with Ramona, walks into the room and snuggles next to her on the couch. "I have had good luck with some of the kids—you know I helped Jacob get toilet trained when he was eleven. But it's because I'm not his mother that I can do a lot of it. Ignoring a tantrum doesn't rip my heart out."

Our settlement comes through. They fund a yearly use-it-or-lose-it annuity that will cover a long-term placement and all of his medical bills.

We tell the state they will not need to fund Porter's placement and a week later we hear that the state will support Porter living with Ramona. Brian and I meet for coffee to make a decision.

"I don't want him to move out, but I can't do it. Obviously I can't keep him safe," I confess.

Our family is shrinking. Soon the group of five will be down to three. I can't picture the future when the weight of the present is suffocating me.

We agree that we can't do it together or alone. We agree it is best for everyone to have Porter move in with Ramona. But it isn't that simple. While I know in my heart that we are doing the right thing, I have never felt so guilty in my life.

Porter has his first trial overnight three weeks later. Ramona picks him up, and he yells, "Bye, Mommy," as she leads him by the hand to the driveway. I see his helmet through the back window of the car as she drives off.

I sit on the couch after they leave, holding a sweatshirt of his and crying, not moving until my legs are stiff. When the sun is completely down, I call Ramona.

"How is he doing?" I ask.

"I know this is hard to hear, Sarah," she says, "but he hasn't asked for you at all. It's not like how it would be for one of your other kids being away from home. You have to believe me when I say that it's good he is responding this way."

Porter moves in with Ramona soon after that, visiting us on weekends.

The following summer, Ramona and I take Porter, Tyler, and Jackson to a rented cabin. After a day of swimming, we put Porter in the tub and I sit on the floor next to Ramona as we give him a bath. I trickle water on his head and wash his hair while Ramona scrubs his feet one at a time. Porter claps his hands as we do it and says, "Hi, Mommy."

In unison, we both say hello back.

EPILOGUE

21 YEARS

"Deep down, we know that when we step back, breathe, allow our agitation to settle, and simply start paying attention, we often see new possibilities in situations that once seem intractable . . . only in this contemplative state are we able to touch the truth . . ."

— Parker Palmer, *The Politics of the Brokenhearted*

Porter is on a gurney at Minneapolis Children's Hospital. He is now twenty-one years old, as they take patients until they are twenty-two. He lies on a bed and his hairy legs stick off the end. I can see them since they cut off his clothes in the ambulance. He's had a seizure and was delivered here by ambulance. His helmet rests on a chair beside him. The curtain to our exam room is open and people hurry in and out. The doctor whispers to the nurse and the nurse gets on the phone.

The seizure won't stop. Not in the ambulance ride over. Not in the ER after three doses of Valium. Not when they add medications to the medications to calm him down. It only stops when everything stops, even his breathing. The seizure has sucked the life out of him.

The doctor moves me out of the way and yells for help. People arrive out of nowhere. They are coming from other rooms and upstairs. Someone in blue scrubs down the hall gives him CPR. Even the doctor looks scared.

They need to move him to a special room. The doctor tells me this and doesn't wait for my reply; they are gone. The nurse grabs his chart, his helmet, his clothes. He is carted away in pieces. Time passes quickly but feels very slow. They are in the resuscitation room and the doctor appears. He says Porter is doing well. Doing well means he isn't dead.

"Porter, it's Mom, can you say something?" I ask. Click. Porter opens his eyes, first one, then the other. Click.

"Can you say something?" I repeat.

Porter smiles. "I want Chicken McNuggets."

Pause. The doctor laughs. "That's a first."

Porter is the best-adjusted person I know. What is remarkable about this is that for all of his medical issues and disabilities, he is happy.

When he was fifteen, he joined the Miracle League baseball team. This is a team of kids with disabilities and each player is partnered with a non-disabled peer. You know it is a different league since no one keeps score. Everyone gets to bat and run the bases whether or not the ball is actually hit.

Shortly after Porter's case was settled, the Vaccine Injury Compensation Program engaged a consultant to create a publicity plan for the court system in Washington, DC. The idea was that clinicians and parents were largely unaware of the special court system to compensate vaccine injuries. The strategists were paid over a quarter of a million dollars and delivered a thorough outreach program to inform health care workers and parents about the fund. Few of the suggestions were implemented.

Porter receives the first payment for his care seven years after we file his case. The settlement covers his care at Ramona's and co-pays for his medications, hospital stays, and ambulance rides. It allots no money for the diapers he wears as an adult.

In 2013, a group of researchers surveyed the diagnoses of children the vaccine court conceded were injured due to immunizations; 50 percent of the children had autism.

Although the government pays for Porter's care, no one has ever requested that he participate in a study looking at what may be different about Porter and the other affected people who won their lawsuits.

No one from the government has ever reached out to ask how he is doing. No government researcher ever followed up to study why he reacted as he did to the vaccine.

Despite it all or because of it, Porter imprints the lives of everyone around him. He outgrew his hyperactivity and his life today centers around puzzles and *Winnie the Pooh* videos and days at the sheltered workshop.

He lives in the present and accepts the moment. There *is* something different about him. Earlier this week, I sat with him in the living room stacking LEGOs into a rickety tower.

"Good job, Mommy!" he cheered, when I placed the last piece.

He knocked it down and started over. A moment later, he looked at me and smiled. "I hear the angels sing," he said.

I smiled too.

I know he does.

ACKNOWLEDGMENTS

I want to thank Brian for being an amazing coparent and father before and after our divorce. I also am eternally grateful to my other coparent, Ramona. Thank you Tyler for your love and strength. You teach me a lot. Porter is lucky to have you as his favorite person on this planet. Thank you to Jackson and Noah (born after these events) for being incredible parts of this village-like family. To my new children, Samantha and Ben: Welcome to the family. Thanks to my higher power for keeping the wheels on the bus.

I wouldn't be the person I am without my father, William Bridges. Thanks for the guidance and thanks for the genes. My mother's doggedness helped us find the path to the vaccine court. Katherine; You are amazing and made the case possible. Life wouldn't be livable without the women in my life: Nina, Suzy, MJ, Susan, Leah, Jill, and Kate. Thank you to David Rowell of the *Washington Post* who first edited my essay on Porter. We miss you, Kathy Rich. Thank you for sending that first piece to the *Post*. Endless gratitude to Lou and the Skyhorse team for making this possible and Krishan for the guidance.

Finally, thank you to my husband, Grant. You've taught me about resilience and helped me create our family of eight. I love you.